THE LIFEWAVE PATCH BIBLE
[8 in 1]

Master the Art of Phototherapy to Enhance Healing, Boost Energy, Relieve Pain, Improve Sleep, and Transform Your Health Naturally

Sophia Raynor

Table of Contents

Introduction

Brief History and Development of Lifewave Patches

Lifewave patches may seem like a modern marvel, but their story traces back to motivated minds and scientific exploration. Back in the early 2000s, a visionary named David Schmidt laid the groundwork. Schmidt, working in fields related to energy and chemistry, embarked on a quest to find a natural yet effective way to boost human energy and wellness.

He began by exploring ways to improve human performance for military applications, focusing on optimizing the body's natural energy based on various research inputs. This quest led him to invent what we now know as Lifewave patches—a tool that takes advantage of phototherapy, using light waves naturally emitted by our bodies.

Initially launched around 2004, these patches were something quite different from what's on the market now. They were simplistic, designed primarily to elevate energy levels without introducing any substances into the body. The technology focused on enhancing cellular communication using a technique rooted in photobiomodulation.

Here's where things get interesting—how it works! Inside each patch is a lattice of organic nanocrystals that are designed to reflect specific wavelengths of light when placed on the skin. Think of it like dialing into the correct radio frequency; these reflected light waves communicate with our body's cells to produce specific health outcomes. Fascinating, right?

Lifewave's journey didn't stall at just one type of patch. Over time, research and customer feedback spurred diversification into multiple patch products, each addressing different wellness goals. For example:

1. **Energy Enhancer (2004):** Kickstarted Lifewave's introduction into the world by aiming at boosting stamina and endurance.
2. **IceWave (2006):** Targeted pain relief without drugs or chemicals.

3. **Y-Age System:** Comprising three patches—Glutathione (2008), Carnosine (2008), and Aeon (2011)—these focus on anti-aging and overall longevity.

4. **Silent Nights (2010):** Optimizing sleep cycles was never this simple; wear one of these patches for improved restful sleep.

5. **SP6 Complete (2011):** Went after appetite control and overall weight management.

Recently they've unveiled X39 (2019), which has been receiving lots of attention due to claims about its anti-aging benefits. This patch supposedly activates stem cells for wound healing and reducing inflammation—certainly innovative!

The popularity rise can be attributed both to personal testimonies and scientific backing that comprise clinical studies demonstrating significant improvement in various health markers upon usage. As the brand expanded globally, alignment with regulations across countries posed some challenges but also expanded consumer trust as they adhered strictly to guidelines ensuring product safety and efficacy.

David Schmidt: The Man Behind LifeWave

David Schmidt, the visionary founder and CEO of LifeWave, is an inventor at heart, driven by a passion for creativity and innovation. Over the past two decades, he has transformed LifeWave from a humble patch company into a pioneering life technology company, aiming to improve life holistically for both humans and the environment. With 139 patents—and counting—David's inventive spirit shows no signs of slowing down.

When David started LifeWave, he had no prior experience in direct selling. However, after witnessing the transformative potential of his technology, his perspective shifted. He realized the immense opportunity in combining his innovative products with network marketing. Thus, LifeWave was born with three initial offerings: patches designed to enhance energy levels, relieve discomfort, and improve sleep—all utilizing light to unlock the body's natural healing capabilities[1].

This was just the beginning. In 2006, David launched new products that used light to synthesize peptides in the body, focusing on anti-aging and performance improvement. By the late 2000s, LifeWave took another giant leap by investing over $4 million into stem cell research and regenerative medicine. This substantial investment produced over 70 global patents and introduced a groundbreaking method of using light to activate stem cells.

2018 marked a pivotal year for LifeWave when they released this innovative product to market. The results were astonishing: robust testimonials from users and impressive outcomes from lab testing and clinical studies fueled soaring growth. From $23 million in sales in 2018 to a staggering $400 million in 2021, David's commitment to innovation proved incredibly fruitful.

LifeWave's remarkable rise is not just about numbers—it's a testament to David's dreams and determination. Now available in 80 countries with 700,000 brand partners globally, David envisions an even brighter future for LifeWave. As the company celebrates its 20th anniversary in the industry, it continues to evolve its offerings significantly.

Later this year, LifeWave plans another major shift from health technology towards becoming a life technology company. This transition includes developing environmentally friendly products aimed at agriculture and power generation—innovations designed not only to enhance quality of life but also promote sustainability.

To David Schmidt and his relentless pursuit of progress: whether it's through expanding technological horizons or uplifting lives across diverse spheres—both human and environmental—his journey thus far has laid a solid foundation for achieving even grander aspirations tomorrow.

Purpose Of This Book and What to Expect

We've all come across various health trends and fads that promise miraculous results but often fall short. LifeWave Patches, however, stand on a solid foundation of science and innovation. Their technology taps into the principles of phototherapy—a method that uses light to enhance your body's natural healing ability. The purpose of this book is to demystify LifeWave Patches and offer you clear, factual insights into how they work and how they can highly enhance your quality of life.

So, what can you expect to learn from reading this book? We've structured it in a way that's both comprehensive and easy to digest, covering multiple aspects that contribute to an informed understanding:

1. **Roots in Phototherapy:** Understanding the broader context of phototherapy helps grasp why LifeWave is effective. The book delves into its history, types, and scientific basis.

2. **Science Simplified:** Get ready for some down-to-earth explanations about how these patches work. We'll cover their workings, ingredients, and comparisons with other methods without burdening you with jargon.

3. **Practical Know-How:** When it comes time to use these patches, placement matters! You'll learn effective strategies for using them—when and where for maximum results—in a straightforward manner.

4. **Health Smorgasbord:** Discover how these patches can aid in relieving pain, boosting energy levels, enhancing sleep patterns, improving mental focus, and supporting your immune function.

5. **Real-Life Proofs:** Real-life case studies offer insights into transformations made possible by these tiny patches across varied user experiences. You'll hear from athletes and see clinical evidence documenting measurable outcomes.

6. **Common Pitfalls and How to Avoid Them:** We're also covering common challenges such as discomfort or misuse, offering solutions based on feedback from users who've been down this road before you.

7. **Future Forecasting:** And if you're curious about what's next for LifeWave? We've sprinkled some advanced insights on upcoming research and future patch developments throughout the text.

"THE LIFEWAVE PATCH BIBLE" is more than just an educational resource; it's a companion guide that empowers you toward informed self-care decisions by utilizing cutting-edge therapies simply and effectively. By engaging deeply with what each section offers, you'll be better prepared not only to use LifeWave patches but also to appreciate how innovations like these are shaping modern health practices.

Download Here your BONUSES!

BOOK 1

Introduction to Phototherapy

History Of Phototherapy

You might be surprised to know that civilizations like the Egyptians, Greeks, and Romans were already harnessing sunlight for healing purposes. The Egyptians were particularly fond of *heliotherapy*, which simply means therapy with natural sunlight[2]. They believed it could treat a range of ailments from skin diseases to fatigue. It turns out they were onto something because scientists now know sunlight prompts our bodies to produce vitamin D, improve mood, and strengthen bones.

Fast forward to the 19th century and we enter a time where scientific exploration took interest in this age-old practice. **Niels Ryberg Finsen** is a big name here; he was a physician from Denmark who is recognized as one of the pioneers in modern phototherapy. Around the late 1800s, Finsen developed an ultraviolet lamp which became famous for treating lupus vulgaris, a form of skin tuberculosis[3]. This was revolutionary and earned him a Nobel Prize in Medicine in 1903. This was a major step in recognizing light as an effective treatment. It was like the world was finally waking up to the idea that light could be more than just something that keeps us company during the day.

As we moved into the 20th century, phototherapy gained even more traction. By the 1920s, doctors were using ultraviolet light to treat various ailments, including skin disorders like psoriasis and eczema. It became a common practice in dermatology clinics. The idea was pretty simple: exposure to certain wavelengths of light could trigger healing processes in the body.

In the 1960s, laser technology began to emerge, and that changed the game for phototherapy. Researchers discovered that specific frequencies of laser light could penetrate deeper into tissues, making them even more effective for healing. This advancement opened the door to treating a wider range of issues, from chronic pain to post-surgery recovery.

As we entered the 21st century, the popularity of phototherapy soared. It became apparent that using light was not just effective but also non-invasive. Many people started looking for alternative treatments that didn't involve heavy medications or surgeries, and phototherapy fit the bill perfectly.

The interesting part about phototherapy is that it's not just limited to treating skin conditions. Many practitioners have also explored its benefits for mental health, seasonal affective disorder (SAD), and even as a way to improve sleep quality. As someone who loves digging into health and wellness topics, I find it fascinating how versatile phototherapy can be.

Today, phototherapy is a well-established field, and many practitioners offer it as part of a holistic approach to health. Whether you're dealing with skin issues, chronic pain, or just looking for a natural way to enhance your overall well-being, phototherapy might be a great option for you.

Science Behind Healing Light

Light is a natural part of our world; it influences countless biological processes in both plants and animals. But here's the kicker—light can also assist in healing our bodies. It sounds almost magical, but there's solid science backing it up.

Phototherapy involves various types of light like visible light, infrared light, and ultraviolet light being applied to our skin. When these light waves interact with our cells, they can help stimulate different biological processes. Let me share an example you might be familiar with: **sunlight**! You know how after some sun exposure, your body starts producing Vitamin D? That's because UVB rays from the sun help convert cholesterol in your skin into Vitamin D3—a crucial vitamin for bone health and immune function.

Similarly, different forms of light used in phototherapy can trigger responses that are super beneficial for human health. Now here's an interesting tidbit: not all types of phototherapy involve the same kind of light or produce identical effects. Various therapies use specific wavelengths tailored for particular purposes.

So, what's going on at a cellular level? Our cells have special components called **"chromophores,"** which are like tiny light receptors. When light hits these chromophores, it triggers a series of chemical reactions that can lead to healing. This is because light can increase energy production in our cells, helping them repair and regenerate more effectively. This absorption can lead to multiple positive effects based on wavelength and intensity. For example:

WAVELENGTH	TYPE OF LIGHT	HEALTH BENEFITS
400-450 nm	Blue Light	Reduces acne, improves mood
450-495 nm	Cyan Light	Reduces inflammation, promotes wound healing
495-570 nm	Green Light	Helps with skin issues, improves skin tone

570-590 nm	Yellow Light	Enhances mood, reduces anxiety
590-620 nm	Orange Light	Boosts immune function
620-750 nm	Red Light	Stimulates collagen production, reduces pain
750-1000 nm	Near-Infrared Light	Penetrates deeply, aids muscle recovery, reduces inflammation

Another great aspect about phototherapy—it's non-invasive! No needles or pills required; just natural restoration using targeted sources of healing frequencies from lights responsibly designed by experts who understand medicine well enough not neglect their professionalism over casual chats like ours today.

Different Types of Phototherapy

Phototherapy describes various treatments that use light to address health concerns. What's interesting is that the type of phototherapy depends greatly on what we're trying to treat.

1 **Bili Lights**: One of the most well-known applications of phototherapy is in the treatment of *neonatal jaundice*, a common condition in newborns characterized by elevated levels of bilirubin in the bloodstream[3]. Bili lights, which emit a specific wavelength of fluorescent light, are utilized to break down bilirubin in the infant's skin[5]. This non-invasive treatment effectively lowers bilirubin levels and helps prevent potential complications, such as kernicterus, a serious neurological condition. The use of bili lights exemplifies how targeted light therapy can dramatically improve health outcomes for vulnerable populations.

2. **Bright Light Therapy**: Nowadays, many individuals struggle with mood and sleep disorders, particularly seasonal affective disorder (SAD) and insomnia. Bright light therapy offers a solution by using lightboxes that mimic natural sunlight[6]. These devices emit bright light at specific intensities and wavelengths to influence circadian rhythms and boost serotonin production. By exposing individuals to bright light, this therapy can alleviate symptoms of depression, improve sleep quality, and promote overall well-being. Bright light therapy has become increasingly popular as a natural, drug-free alternative for managing mood-related issues.

3. **Broadband UVB**: Broadband ultraviolet-B (UVB) therapy is an effective treatment primarily used for skin conditions such as psoriasis, eczema, and vitiligo[7]. This treatment utilizes a wide

range of UVB rays, which are present in natural sunlight but are not visible to the human eye. By exposing the skin to these UVB rays, the therapy helps to reduce inflammation and slow down the rapid skin cell growth that characterizes many dermatological conditions. While beneficial, it is important for patients to be monitored during treatment, as excessive exposure to UVB rays can lead to skin damage.

4. **Narrowband UVB**: Narrowband UVB therapy is a more refined approach that uses a specific and narrower wavelength of UVB light. This method has become the most common type of light therapy used today for treating skin conditions[8]. The more focused beam allows for more precise targeting of affected areas, leading to effective results with potentially fewer side effects compared to broadband UVB. Narrowband UVB has gained popularity for its ability to provide relief with shorter treatment sessions, making it a convenient choice for many patients suffering from chronic skin ailments.

5. **PUVA Therapy**: Psoralen ultraviolet-A, or PUVA, represents a more complex type of phototherapy that combines UVA light with a plant-derived chemical called psoralen[9]. Psoralen is applied to the skin prior to exposure to UVA light, enhancing the skin's sensitivity to the light and allowing for a more potent therapeutic effect. PUVA is particularly effective in treating severe skin conditions such as psoriasis and certain types of eczema. Due to its strength, this therapy is generally reserved for cases that have not responded to other treatments, and patients require careful monitoring throughout the process.

TYPE	PRIMARY USE	LIGHT TYPE
Bili Lights	Newborn Jaundice	Fluorescent lights
Bright Light Therapy	Mood and Sleep Disorders	Lightbox mimicking natural sunlight
Broadband UVB	Skin Conditions (e.g., psoriasis)	Ultraviolet-B
Narrowband UVB	Common Skin Conditions (e.g., psoriasis)	Intense Ultraviolet-B
PUVA	Severe Skin Conditions (e.g., severe psoriasis)	Ultraviolet-A + Psoralen

How Patches Fit into Phototherapy

LifeWave patches are these small, adhesive patches that you apply to your skin. They work by using light, heat, and your body's own energy to promote healing and boost energy levels. You might be thinking, *"Wait, how does that relate to phototherapy?"* Well, phototherapy focuses on using light to treat various conditions, and patches harness the power of light in a unique way.

Patches are designed to reflect light back into your body. When you place a patch on your skin, it interacts with your body's natural heat and creates a subtle light frequency. This frequency can stimulate various biological responses, promoting healing and wellness without any invasive procedures[10].

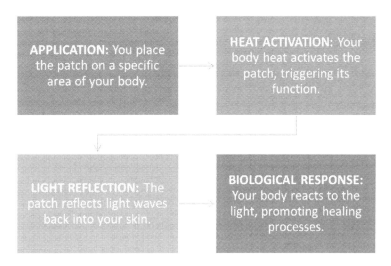

Now that we have a basic understanding, let's talk about the benefits of using patches in the context of phototherapy.

1. **Local Treatment:** Patches can be applied directly to the area that needs attention. For example, if you have discomfort in your back, you can place a patch right where it hurts. This localized approach often means quicker relief.

2. **Non-Invasive:** Unlike some traditional phototherapy treatments that may require specialized equipment or procedures, patches are easy to use and do not require a doctor's visit. You can apply them in the comfort of your home.

3. **Portability:** Patches are small and discreet. You can take them anywhere, which means you can maintain your wellness routine even while traveling or on the go.

4. **No Side Effects:** Since patches use your body's own energy and light, they generally have minimal to no side effects. This is a huge advantage compared to some medications that can come with a laundry list of adverse effects.

5. **Simplicity:** Applying a patch is simple. There are no complicated instructions or dosages to remember. You simply place it, and you're good to go!

One of the great things about patches is that they can easily fit into your existing wellness routine. Whether you're practicing yoga, meditating, or even just enjoying a quiet evening at home, you can incorporate the patches without any hassle.

You might find that combining patches with other therapies enhances your overall results. For instance, using a patch while you're relaxing in a warm bath can create a soothing experience while promoting healing. Just make sure to pay attention to how your body responds and adjust as needed.

BOOK 2

Understanding LifeWave Patches

How Lifewave Patches Work

Lifewave patches are designed to utilize the light emitted naturally by our bodies. They cleverly interact with this light through organic nanocrystals embedded in each patch. These unique formations are not just any crystals; they're proprietary and patented designs that have been meticulously crafted.

Each patch comprises specific combinations of amino acids, water, stabilized oxygen, sugars, and salts which together form distinct crystal lattice structures. Due to these structural differences, each variety of patch reflects a unique light frequency back into the body[11]. When this happens, specific beneficial peptides are produced within our systems.

What's mind-blowing is how these patches target peptides that activate various meridian pathways within us. Now, why is this important? Meridians are like highways in our bodies that facilitate energy flow. By influencing them positively through peptide activation, Lifewave patches aid in enhancing our health over the long term.

They're completely non-invasive—meaning nothing actually enters your body during their use! They're latex-free, non-transdermal, and contain zero drugs or chemicals. So, if you're on any medication, no worries there—the patches won't interfere because they don't introduce foreign substances into your body. Their sole function is to reflect back the natural wavelengths your body emits.

While Lifewave patches are standalone marvels, incorporating them into a healthy lifestyle amplifies their effects even more! Whether you're mindful eating, maintaining a regular exercise routine, or practicing stress-relief techniques, combining these life choices with the use of Lifewave can only enhance your overall well-being.

Types of LifeWave Patches

If you're keen on exploring all the different patches available and what they can do for you, you're in the right place. Below are the types of LifeWave patches, helping you understand what each can do so you can choose the one that fits your needs best[12].

Energy Enhancer: Natural Energy

Ever feel like you need a boost but want to avoid caffeine or other stimulants? The Energy Enhancer patch is your solution. Supporting beta-oxidation—a process where fat is converted into energy—this patch naturally boosts cellular energy production. Clinically proven to increase endurance and overall energy levels without drugs or stimulants, it's a must-have for those with a busy lifestyle or anyone seeking a performance boost[13].

Glutathione: Detox

For those needing detoxification support, the Glutathione patch is indispensable. Known as the body's master antioxidant, glutathione aids organ and cellular detoxification efficiently. This patch notably boosts glutathione levels in the body by about 300% within 24 hours. Use it one to three times weekly for optimal benefits without overwhelming your system.

IceWave: Pain Relief

Chronic pain can be debilitating and hinders everyday activities. Enter IceWave—designed with two patches allowing users to pinpoint and alleviate pain dynamically. Like other LifeWave patches, it's non-transdermal with zero drugs involved—it's absolutely safe with no risk of addiction or harmful side effects. Whether you're dealing with acute injuries or persistent aches, IceWave offers a viable alternative.

Silent Nights: Sleep Improvement

Getting quality sleep is crucial yet challenging for many people today. Silent Nights assists your body in producing melatonin—essential for sleep regulation—without introducing external chemicals or drugs. Dr. Norm Shealy's study revealed that Silent Nights improved sleep quality and length by up to 60%, meaning more restful nights are just a patch away[14].

SP6: Cravings Control

Eating habits can be hard to manage, especially when faced with intense cravings or hunger pangs. SP6 patches assist users in controlling those compelling urges naturally by stimulating the SP6 acupressure point in the body. This stimulation helps moderate appetite and suppresses cravings effectively without resorting to any form of medication or stimulant—making it an excellent companion for weight management journeys.

X39: The Repair Patch

The X39 patch is all about cellular repair and stem cell activation. By elevating GHK-Cu levels, it aids in rejuvenating and resetting over 4,000 genes for a healthier state. You'll find it helpful for wound healing, reducing inflammatory pain, and improving skin, hair, and nail health. Plus, it supports better energy levels and sleep quality while contributing to hormonal balance and brain health, which can ease depression and anxiety.

X49: Performance Enhancer

If you're looking to boost physical performance, the X49 patch is your go-to option. It elevates AHK-Cu, enhancing alanine production to improve strength, stamina, and recovery. Enhanced cardiovascular health and cognitive functions also come along with increased bone density and muscle gain. Interestingly, anecdotal evidence suggests that it helps the body withstand electromagnetic frequencies (EMF) better.

AEON: Stress & Inflammation Relief

Need some 'zen' time? AEON is considered an anti-aging patch due to its ability to reduce stress-related markers such as cortisol. Known as the *"happy"* patch, it raises SOD levels for improved stress management—imagine consuming 30 cups of Royal Jelly! It balances the autonomic nervous system while aiding hormonal production stability.

ALAVIDA: For Skin Beauty

Alavida is perfect for anyone looking to improve skin health from within. This patch elevates epithalamin or epithalon, peptides known for their cellular anti-aging benefits. By enhancing chromosome repair, Alavida reduces fine lines and wrinkles, brightens the complexion, and evens out skin tone. If you want your skin to glow naturally without invasive treatments, Alavida is a top choice.

Carnosine: Brain & Circulatory Health

Your brain and heart deserve the best care, which is precisely what the Carnosine patch offers. It increases carnosine production in your body—a dipeptide that protects brain function and impedes aging effects by improving antioxidation of organs. Found in the brain, heart, and muscles, carnosine enhances cognitive function, helps stave off mental decline, and supports visual health. It's also beneficial for athletes as it boosts strength, stamina, and flexibility.

One great thing about LifeWave patches is how they cater to different needs specifically yet seamlessly work together if you decide to combine them based on personal objectives or lifestyle requirements.

Key Ingredients of Lifewave Patches

Now, you might be wondering what's inside these small, seemingly simple patches? It's an excellent question because Lifewave patches work quite differently from your typical cream or pill. They don't actually put any substances into your body; rather, they're made up of organic stuff that interacts with your body's energy.

The magic of Lifewave patches lies in their unique blend of specific ingredients encased within layers that are meant to reflect certain light wavelengths. The core components are amino acids, sugars, salt, water, and stabilized oxygen[15]. Yup, that's right—simple yet powerful elements! When combined with nanotechnology that communicates with our body's infrared light and heat, they create a sort of symphony for stimulating specific therapeutic responses.

1. **Amino Acids:** These are the building blocks of proteins and important in nearly every biological process. In Lifewave patches, they help form the crystal lattice structure that makes phototherapy with light so effective at communicating with your body.
2. **Water:** It's not just any ordinary water but rather structured for stability and function within the patch. Water acts as a medium or carrier in many cellular processes and helps facilitate energy transfer within the patch.

3. **Stabilized Oxygen:** This ingredient is all about enhancing your body's natural ability to utilize oxygen more efficiently. By incorporating stabilized oxygen into the patch's design, there's an increased potential for energy production in the cells.

4. **Sugars:** These aren't just sweet for taste; they're molecularly essential in forming stable crystals within the patch. They interact uniquely to enhance functionality without adding calories to your wellness routine!

5. **Salts**: Different types of salts are essential for establishing an effective crystal lattice structure within each patch. They ensure that every signal sent to your body is clear and unimpeded.

INGREDIENT	ROLE IN PATCHES
Amino Acids	Forming protein structures and building crystal lattices
Water	Functions as a medium/carrier for energy transfer
Stabilized Oxygen	Enhances cellular energy utilization
Sugars	Helps form stable crystal structures
Salts	Important for signal clarity and stability

Once applied to our skin, these components interact with our body's heat—and our natural infra-red light—to start the phototherapy process we talked about earlier without adding anything invasive or chemical-filled into our system. What makes them especially interesting is that they're non-transdermal; that means they don't release anything through the skin—it's all about energetic interaction. Isn't it cool how something seemingly minuscule can provide connection pathways for our bodies to naturally perform at their best?

Lifewave ensures that each patch leads to distinct effects based on their unique proportions and combinations amongst these ingredients. This mixture ensures compatibility with your body's natural processes without introducing foreign substances.

The Science and Technology Behind

Lifewave patches are innovative tools designed to improve health and well-being by using the body's natural energy fields. They are non-invasive and drug-free, making them a great alternative for those looking for natural approaches. So, how do these patches actually work?

Lifewave patches utilize phototherapy, a technology that's been around for ages. Here's the cool part: our bodies respond to different wavelengths of light in various ways. For example, some wavelengths can prompt physical changes by inducing responses like reducing inflammation or increasing energy production at the cellular level.

Let's look at what happens with the Lifewave Energy Enhancer patch. When applied, the patch reflects certain infrared and visible light back into the skin. This particular wavelength of light has been shown to increase ATP production in cells, which is like getting a shot of energy right where you need it! ATP (adenosine triphosphate) is essentially the body's fuel—more ATP means more energy for physical activities.

Moreover, folks often wonder if there's any science backing up these claims. Lifewave has conducted several clinical studies on their patches that demonstrate various benefits such as increased stamina and pain relief. These studies typically test against placebo groups to ensure the results are legitimate.

Another notable patch is the IceWave patch designed for pain relief. This patch works similarly by modifying how your body processes pain signals through changes in cellular activities driven by reflected light waves. It's fascinating because instead of masking pain like traditional medications might do, these patches aim to address it naturally.

Now let's talk benefits! Users report feeling more energetic and experiencing less pain without having to ingest anything—this is advantageous for people who are cautious about over-the-counter medication use or have sensitivities to certain substances.

Lifewave patches can potentially boost well-being by harnessing phototherapy without unwanted side effects typically associated with pharmacological solutions.

Lifewave Patches Comparisons with Other Methods

If you're exploring ways to improve your health, you've probably come across a variety of options, from supplements to physical therapies. Here, we'll break down Lifewave patches compared to some traditional and alternative methods, so you can see how they measure up.

LifeWave Patches vs. Traditional Medications

When most people think about pain relief or wellness methods, they often turn to traditional medications. These can include over-the-counter options like ibuprofen or prescription painkillers. While these can offer quick relief, they often come with a list of potential side effects, including stomach issues, drowsiness, and even dependency if used long-term.

Unlike traditional medications, LifeWave patches are non-invasive and have no known side effects. They work by stimulating specific points on the body to promote natural healing. This means you can find relief without the risks associated with drugs. Plus, with LifeWave, you're not masking the problem; you're encouraging your body to heal itself.

FEATURE	TRADITIONAL MEDICATIONS	LIFEWAVE PATCHES
Side Effects	Often present	None reported
Method of Use	Oral or injectable	Stick-on patches
Dependency Risk	High	None
Duration of Effects	Short-lived	Varies, can be longer
Cost	Varies	Affordable

LifeWave Patches vs. Acupuncture

Acupuncture involves inserting thin needles into specific points on the body. Many people find acupuncture effective for pain relief, stress reduction, and overall wellness. The downside? It requires visiting a trained professional, which can be time-consuming and potentially costly.

With LifeWave, you get the benefits of similar point stimulation without the needles or the need for appointments. You can use the patches at home whenever you need them, giving you much more flexibility and convenience. Plus, they're easy to apply and remove, making them a great option if you're busy or just don't like needles.

FEATURE	ACUPUNCTURE	LIFEWAVE PATCHES
Professional Needed	Yes	No
Pain Level	Mild discomfort	No discomfort
Flexibility	Appointment-based	Anytime, anywhere
Cost	Can be high	Affordable
Learning Curve	Requires training	Simple to use

LifeWave Patches vs. Physical Therapy

Physical Therapy involves working with a trained therapist to regain movement, strength, and function. While physical therapy can be very effective, it often requires a significant time commitment and can be quite expensive. Sessions may range from 30 minutes to an hour, several times a week.

In contrast, LifeWave patches can complement physical therapy or stand alone as a more accessible option. You can use the patches to enhance your healing process without the need for frequent visits. Many users find that patches help relieve pain and inflammation, allowing them to engage in physical therapy more effectively.

FEATURE	PHYSICAL THERAPY	LIFEWAVE PATCHES
Professional Needed	Yes	No
Time Commitment	High	Minimal
Cost	Often expensive	Affordable
Flexibility	Scheduled sessions	Anytime, anywhere
Personalization	Tailored by therapist	General application

As you can see, LifeWave patches offer a unique and convenient option for those looking to enhance their healing journey. They eliminate many of the drawbacks associated with traditional medications, acupuncture, and physical therapy. If you're looking for a simple, effective way to improve your overall well-being, LifeWave patches are worth considering.

Safety and Efficacy

When it comes to health and wellness products, two words that always pop up are "safety" and "efficacy." Nobody wants to use something that could cause harm, and everyone wants to see results, right? The primary concerns often revolve around potential side effects, allergies, and interactions with other treatments or medications. For the LifeWave patches, numerous studies have been conducted to evaluate these aspects.

1. **Non-Invasive Nature:** LifeWave patches are designed to be non-invasive. This means they don't penetrate the skin or require needles, making them a safe option for most people.
2. **Hypoallergenic Materials**: The patches are made from materials that have been tested for skin compatibility. This helps reduce the risk of allergic reactions.
3. **No Drugs or Chemicals:** One of the standout features of LifeWave patches is that they don't contain any drugs or chemicals. Instead, they work by utilizing light therapy principles, which means you're not putting anything harmful into your body.

When we talk about efficacy, we're really interested in whether the patches do what they claim to do. Studies and user testimonials provide valuable insights into how effective the patches can be. Here's a summary of what the research indicates:

1. **Pain Relief:** Many users report significant reductions in pain levels after using the patches. Clinical studies have shown that the patches can help alleviate discomfort, making everyday tasks much easier.
2. **Improved Sleep:** Sleep issues are common nowadays. Many people have found that using specific patches can help them achieve better quality sleep. Research supports this, indicating that users often experience improved sleep patterns.
3. **Enhanced Energy:** Numerous testimonials highlight increased energy levels after using the patches. People report feeling less fatigued and more focused throughout the day.

FEATURE	SAFETY MEASURES	EFFICACY EVIDENCE
Non-Invasive	No needles or skin penetration	Users report reduced pain levels
Hypoallergenic	Tested for skin compatibility	Improved sleep quality reported
Drug-Free	No harmful chemicals involved	Increased energy and focus

While research is essential, user experiences often tell a compelling story. Many people have shared how the patches have positively impacted their lives. It's not just about studies; real-world applications showcase their usability.

1. **Testimonials:** Many users rave about how quickly they felt relief from headaches or muscle pain after just a few uses.
2. **Community Feedback:** Online forums and support groups for LifeWave users often highlight personal experiences, providing a sense of community and shared discovery.

Coupled with the growing body of user testimonials and scientific research supporting their effectiveness, it's easy to see why so many people are turning to these patches as a solution for pain relief, sleep improvement, and overall wellness.

BOOK 3
Using Patches Effectively

Placement Mastery

The LifeWave patches are designed to stimulate specific points on your body, much like acupressure or acupuncture, but without the needles. When you place the patches correctly, they can help enhance your body's natural healing processes, boost energy, reduce pain, and improve overall wellness.

When you're deciding where to place your patches, keep these factors in mind:

1. **Specific Ailments:** Depending on what you're trying to address—be it pain, fatigue, or even sleep issues—placement can vary. Certain patches work better for specific issues, so understanding your need will guide you.

2. **Sensitivity:** Everyone's body responds differently. If you feel any discomfort at a particular placement, it's wise to try a different spot.

3. **Comfort:** You want to put the patches in places that won't interfere with your daily activities. Avoid spots that might rub against clothing or get in the way during movement.

PATCH	PLACEMENT AREA	BENEFITS
Energy Enhancer	On the upper chest	Boosts energy and stamina
Ice Wave	Painful area and opposite side	Reduces pain and inflammation
Silent Nights	On the back of the neck or wrists	Improves sleep quality
X39	Below the navel or behind the neck	Promotes healing and rejuvenation
SP6 Complete	On the upper chest	Boosts energy and stamina

Now that you have a basic idea of where to place the patches, let's talk about how to apply them effectively:

1. **Clean Skin:** Make sure the area is clean and dry. This helps the patch stick well and also ensures that nothing interferes with its function.

2. **Press Firmly:** After placing the patch, press down gently but firmly to ensure it adheres properly. You want it to stay in place throughout your day.

3. **Rotate Placements:** If you're using more than one patch or using the same patch for an extended period, it's good to rotate placements. This can help prevent skin irritation and ensure you're getting the most out of your patches.

As you start using the patches, pay attention to how your body responds. Everyone is unique, so what works for one person might not work for another. If you find a certain placement brings amazing results, stick with it. If not, don't hesitate to experiment a little—just keep everything we discussed in mind.

To maximize your experience, consider keeping a simple journal. Write down where you placed the patches, your feelings before and after using them, and any changes you noticed. This will help you identify patterns and discover what works best for you.

Timing for Maximum Results

Timing isn't just about when you start your day. It's about understanding your body's natural rhythms and how the LifeWave patches can work best within those rhythms. Here are some key points to keep in mind:

1. **Morning vs. Evening:** Many people find that applying patches in the morning helps kickstart their day. This is especially true for patches aimed at boosting energy and alertness. On the flip side, some patches are great for relaxation and recovery, which makes evening application ideal. Test it for yourself to see what works best for you.

2. **Duration of Use:** Different patches may have different recommended durations. While some patches are designed for continuous wear throughout the day (like 12 hours), others may be better suited for shorter applications. Always check the guidelines provided with each patch and adjust your timing accordingly.

3. **Activity Levels:** Consider what you're doing throughout your day. If you're planning a workout or an intense activity, applying a patch that supports energy and stamina before your session can enhance your performance. Similarly, using patches that promote recovery post-exercise can help your body bounce back faster.

TIME OF DAY	RECOMMENDED PATCHES	PURPOSE
Morning	Energy patches	Kickstart your day and boost alertness
Midday	Stress relief patches	Keep calm and focused
Evening	Restorative patches	Promote relaxation and recovery
Pre-Workout	Performance enhancement patches	Maximize workout efficiency
Post-Workout	Recovery patches	Aid muscle recovery

Everyone reacts differently to patches and their application times. Keep a simple journal or notes on how you feel with different patches at different times of the day. Track your energy levels, mood, and any changes you notice. This can help you find the perfect timing routine just for you.

Now, let's touch on something many of us might not think about: our natural body clocks, also known as **circadian rhythms**. These rhythms influence various bodily functions, including sleep, digestion, and even hormonal balance. For example, your body tends to release cortisol, the stress hormone, in the morning, which helps you wake up and feel alert. Using an energy-boosting patch during this time can harmonize with this natural peak in cortisol levels.

On the other hand, melatonin production increases at night, helping prepare your body for sleep. Applying a patch designed to promote relaxation in the evening can support this natural wind-down period.

In the end, the best timing for using LifeWave patches depends on your personal preferences and lifestyle. Don't be afraid to experiment! Try different patches at various times, and see what feels right. You may find that certain patches work wonders in the morning, while others shine in the evening.

Understanding Custom Protocols

Creating custom protocols with LifeWave patches means designing a patching routine that suits your unique needs. It's about listening to your body and responding with the right patch at the right time. Everyone's health journey is different, so having the flexibility to personalize your approach can be truly empowering.

1. **Identify Your Needs:** Clearly defining what you want to achieve. Are you looking to boost energy, improve sleep, relieve pain, or enhance mental clarity? Pinpoint these goals as they will guide your protocol design.

2. **Patch Selection:** Consider which patches align with your goals. For instance:

> *For energy:* Try the Energy Enhancer patches.

> *For sleep improvement:* The Silent Nights patch might be your go-to.

> *For pain relief:* IceWave is a popular choice.

3. **Listen to Feedback from Your Body**: As you try different patches and combinations, pay close attention to how your body responds. You might notice some immediate effects or require more time to gauge changes.

4. **Experimentation and Adjustment:** Don't be afraid to tweak your protocol based on your experiences. You can adjust placement slightly, try different combinations of patches, or modify the times you apply them.

5. **Record the Effects:** Keep a journal of what you notice. Writing down any changes—whether mental, emotional, or physical—can provide valuable insight into what's working and what's not.

Sample Protocols

Below are examples of how some individuals might structure their protocol based on specific goals:

For Daily Energy:

> ➢ Apply the Energy Enhancer patches on specific acupoints first thing in the morning.
> ➢ Adjust placement mid-day if energy begins dipping.

For Improved Sleep:

➢ Use Silent Nights 30 minutes before bedtime.

➢ Pair with relaxation techniques such as deep breathing.

For Pain Relief:

➢ Place IceWave patches directly over or near areas of discomfort.

➢ Use complementary techniques like gentle stretching when possible.

Taking control of your health can be as simple as establishing a routine that addresses your specific wellness goals using LifeWave patches. While these guidelines offer a foundation, remember that there isn't a one-size-fits-all approach—so feel free to create something uniquely yours!

Self-Assessment Worksheet

Step 1: Rate Your Goals

List the specific goals you identified at the start of your LifeWave journey:

1. _____

2. _____

3. _____

For each goal, rate your current satisfaction level using the patches:

GOAL #	CURRENT SATISFACTION (0-10)	NOTES ON PROGRESS OR BARRIERS
1		
2		
3		

Step 2: Evaluate Patch Performance

Reflect on how each type of patch you're using has performed:

1. *For increased energy:* Rate how well the Energy Enhancer patches met your needs on a scale of 0 to 10.
2. *For better sleep:* Rate Silent Nights for helping improve your sleep quality.
3. *For pain relief:* Rate IceWave effectiveness in alleviating discomfort.

PATCH TYPE	PERFORMANCE RATING (0-10)	OBSERVATIONS AND ADJUSTMENTS
Energy Enhancer		
Silent Nights		
IceWave		

Step 3: Analyze Timing and Placement

Check in on whether adjusting patch placement or timing offers improved results:

1. Have you tried varying times for applying them?
2. Have you explored different locations for patch placement?

Record any changes and realized benefits:

CHANGE MADE	RESULT NOTED

Step 4: Overall Satisfaction

End by reflecting on these key questions:

1. Do you feel empowered by managing your own health protocol?
2. Are there areas where you'd like more improvement?

Rate your overall satisfaction with the patch routine: ___ / 10

Based on this self-assessment, consider what tweaks might improve your routine. Remember, experimentation is part of finding what works best for you! Take these insights, adjust as needed, and continue to document your journey. Feel free to revisit this worksheet regularly to track changes over time.

Avoiding Common Errors

These patches have a lot to offer, but like anything new, there are some common mistakes that can hamper your experience. Don't worry, though—we're here to help you handle this smoothly. Below are some of the common errors people make when using Lifewave patches and how you can avoid them[16].

1. **Applying Patches on Dirty Skin**: Make sure your skin is clean before applying the patches. If you apply a patch on dirty or oily skin, it may not adhere properly, and you might not get the full benefits. Just wash the area with soap and water and let it dry completely before applying the patch. It's a small step that can make a big difference!

2. **Overlapping Patches**: LifeWave patches are designed to be placed on specific points on your body. If you're tempted to overlap patches, it might seem like you're maximizing their effect. However, this can actually interfere with how they work. Make sure to place each patch in its designated spot without overlapping them. Check the patch instructions for specific placement guidance.

3. **Forgetting to Rotate Patches**: Using the same patch on the same spot for too long can lead to skin irritation and reduced effectiveness. It's a good idea to rotate your patches daily or as indicated in the instructions. This practice keeps your skin healthy and allows for better absorption of the patch's benefits. Just jot down a reminder on your calendar or phone to help you remember!

4. **Ignoring the Recommended Duration:** Each patch has a recommended duration for how long it should be worn, usually ranging from 8 to 12 hours. Some people think that wearing a patch longer will provide more benefits, but that's not the case. Exceeding the recommended duration can lead to skin irritation or decreased effectiveness. Stick to the guidelines provided, and you'll be just fine!

5. **Not Drinking Enough Water**: When using LifeWave patches, make sure to drink plenty of water. Proper hydration can help your body process the effects of the patches and support overall well-being. Aim for at least 8 cups of water a day, especially when you're using the patches regularly.

6. **Not Paying Attention to Your Body**: Everyone's body reacts differently to patches, so it's essential to listen to what your body is telling you. If you notice any discomfort, irritation, or unusual reactions, it's best to remove the patch and consult a healthcare professional. Trust your instincts and prioritize your health.

7. **Misunderstanding Patch Types**: LifeWave offers a variety of patches, each designed for different purposes. Make sure you're using the right type of patch for what you want to achieve. For example, energy patches are different from pain relief patches. Check the packaging and ensure you're using the right one for your specific needs.

8. **Skipping the Follow-Up**: Using LifeWave patches isn't just a one-and-done deal. Keep a record of how you feel over time. This can help you understand which patches work best for you and how to adjust your routine. It's like having your own personal healing journal. You might even discover patterns or improvements you wouldn't have noticed otherwise.

By keeping these common errors in mind and making simple adjustments, you'll set yourself up for success with LifeWave patches.

Tracking Progress and Consistency

When you start using LifeWave patches, it's easy to get caught up in the excitement and forget to pay attention to how you're feeling over time. By tracking your progress, you can see the positive changes and gains you're making, which helps keep you motivated. Plus, it allows you to adjust your routine if necessary to optimize your experience.

Here are some key elements to keep an eye on while using LifeWave patches:

1. **Symptoms:** Write down your starting symptoms. If you're using patches for pain relief, for instance, note the intensity and frequency of your pain. This will help you gauge how effective the patches are over time.

2. **Energy Levels:** Take note of your overall energy levels. Are you feeling more energetic throughout the day? Are you experiencing fewer energy crashes?

3. **Sleep Quality:** If you're looking to improve your sleep, track how well you sleep. Are you falling asleep faster? Are you waking up feeling more refreshed?

4. **Mood:** Your emotional state is important too. Jot down any noticeable changes in your mood or stress levels. Feeling less anxious or more positive can be a sign that the patches are working for you.

5. **Physical Activity:** If you're using the patches to support recovery from workouts, keep a record of your exercise routine. Are you able to push yourself harder? Are you recovering more quickly?

You can track your progress in several ways. Here are a few methods:

1. **Journaling:** Keep a simple journal where you write down your daily observations. This can be as easy as noting how you feel each day after using the patches.

2. **Apps:** Use health-tracking apps to log your symptoms, energy levels, and other factors. Many apps are user-friendly and allow you to visualize your progress through charts and graphs.

3. **Progress Charts:** Consider creating a simple chart to track your symptoms and progress over time. Here's an example:

DATE	SYMPTOM SEVERITY (1-10)	ENERGY LEVEL (1-10)	SLEEP QUALITY (1-10)	MOOD (1-10)
Day 1	7	4	5	6
Day 7	5	6	6	7
Day 14	3	8	8	8
Day 21	2	9	9	9

This table is just a starting point. You can customize it to fit your preferences. The goal is to make tracking enjoyable and straightforward, not a chore!

Staying Consistent

Now that you know what to track, let's talk about consistency. The benefits of LifeWave patches build up over time, so using them regularly is key.

1. Create a daily routine for applying the patches. Whether it's morning or night, pick a time that works best for you. Consistency is crucial!

2. Use your phone, a calendar, or sticky notes to remind yourself to put on your patches. It's easy to forget, especially when life gets busy.

3. Share your journey with a friend or family member. Sometimes, just having someone to check in with can keep you on track.

4. Acknowledge your progress along the way, no matter how small. This will help maintain your motivation and keep the journey enjoyable.

Tracking your progress and staying consistent with LifeWave patches can make a big difference in your healing journey. By noting changes in your symptoms, energy levels, sleep quality, and mood, you can see how the patches are working for you. Remember, every little detail counts! Stick with it, and don't hesitate to adjust your approach as you learn what works best for you.

BOOK 4

Health Benefits Explored

Relieving Chronic Pain

Chronic pain is something that many of us encounter, and it can often feel like a constant companion that's difficult to shake off. Whether it's that persistent backache or the migraine that just won't quit, finding relief becomes a top priority for those experiencing chronic pain. The Lifewave patches have emerged as a promising tool to offer comfort and ease to individuals grappling with such issues.

Chronic pain persists for weeks, months, or even years and can stem from a variety of conditions like arthritis, fibromyalgia, old injuries, or other underlying health issues. Chronic pain not only affects one's physical well-being but can also take a toll on mental health, making day-to-day life challenging.

IceWave is part of the LifeWave family of patches designed to make your life easier by targeting pain without resorting to medication[17]. Yes, you heard it right! No pills, no creams, and definitely no needles involved. The patches work externally, which means they don't transfer any substance into your body. So, those worried about side effects or potential addiction can breathe easy—IceWave has got you covered.

IceWave comes as a set of two patches that you apply close to the pain area. Why two? Well, this dual patch system lets you target the pain more accurately. You simply place one "*white*" patch on one side of the painful area and the "*tan*" patch directly opposite. This method amplifies its effectiveness by concentrating on specific points that align with traditional energy flow theories.

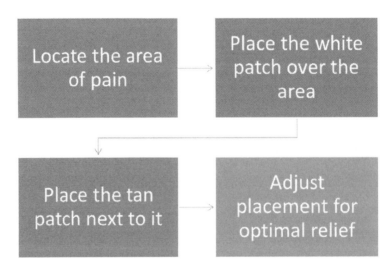

Let's say you've got a nagging lower back problem or an achy knee—IceWave allows customization in placement so that you're not tackling chronic pain blindly. Whether it's an acute injury or that familiar persistent ache, switching up positions depending on current discomfort levels gives you control.

You might wonder how an adhesive patch could possibly alleviate chronic pain just like that. The answer lies in its design and mechanism, which has been reviewed by several users and backed with real success stories. These patches harness specific wavelengths of light (invisible to our eyes) which are thought to stimulate certain points on the body much like acupuncture but without needles.

Now let's address why so many people are adopting IceWave as part of their pain management routine:

1. **Instant Results:** Many users have reported feeling relief within minutes, not hours or days.
2. **Customizable Application:** Based on personal comfort and where pain surfaces.
3. **Everyday Use:** Safe enough for everyday life whether you're running errands or exercising.
4. **Uncomplicated Alternatives:** Instead of relying solely on traditional pain relievers, which might cause long-term harm or side effects, IceWave offers another path.

For anyone dealing with chronic pain, embracing new approaches is often accompanied by skepticism—and rightly so! Attempting new methods can be daunting when dealing with recurring issues requiring incessant management efforts from both sufferer and caregiver alike.

PAIN TYPE	RECOMMENDED PLACEMENT	SUGGESTED DURATION
Back Pain	Lower back area	12 hours per day
Knee Pain	Around the knee cap	8 hours per day
Neck Tension	Base of neck	10 hours per day

Improving Energy Levels

Whether it's powering through your day at work, keeping up with the kids, or just wanting to feel more vibrant, increasing your energy levels can make a huge difference. Energy helps us function physically and mentally. Many factors can affect our energy levels, including stress, diet, sleep, and even the environment. LifeWave patches are designed to naturally support your body's energy systems without the jitters that come from caffeine or other stimulants.

LifeWave patches work by utilizing a unique blend of materials that interact with your body's energy points. When you place a patch on your skin, it helps to stimulate these energy points, promoting better circulation and overall energy flow. This can be particularly useful for those who experience fatigue or a mid-day slump.

There are different types of LifeWave patches that can help with energy. Here are a couple of popular options:

The Energy Enhancer Patch

The Energy Enhancer patch is designed to improve energy flow within the body. Imagine feeling sluggish after lunch or battling through an afternoon slump; that's where this patch can make a real difference. By increasing bioelectrical activity, it helps maintain high energy levels without relying on caffeine or sugar spikes which usually lead to a crash afterward.

What sets the Energy Enhancer apart? It aims to:

1. **Boost Stamina:** Perfect for those who need a little extra pep in their step throughout the day.
2. **Reduce Fatigue:** Ideal if you feel tired but need to continue performing at your best.
3. **Enhance Athletic Performance:** Many athletes use it to support better workout outcomes.

Recent studies have shown users of the patch reported increased performance in physical activities and less feeling of fatigue compared to before they started using it.

The X39 Patch

It's known as a *"jack-of-all-trades"* in the patch world since it's designed to support not only energy enhancement but also overall well-being. Why? Because it encourages your body to activate stem cells which further supports various biological processes.

Here are some specifically targeted benefits:

1. **Rejuvenation:** Users often experience a youthful verve and vitality.
2. **Overall Better Functioning:** With activated stem cells working their magic, your body might just surprise you with how efficiently it starts working.
3. **Increased Physical Activity Recovery:** This means quicker recovery times post-exercise, leaving more time for activities without needing extended downtime.

Many users noticed more sustained energy without jitters or a big crash later on—a common complaint with other energizers like caffeine-based products.

When selecting a patch, consider your specific needs. Are you looking for an energy boost during workouts? The Energy Enhancer patch might be your go-to. If you're after overall support, the X39 could be the answer.

To get the best results from your patches, follow these simple steps:

1. **Clean the Area:** Make sure the skin is clean and dry before applying the patch. This helps ensure good adhesion and effectiveness.
2. **Apply the Patch:** Place the patch on a point where you feel comfortable, such as on the upper arm or below the collarbone. For energy, consider placing it on a spot aligned with your energy channels, like the stomach area.
3. **Wear It:** Keep the patch on for a minimum of 12 hours. You can wear it longer; many people find they benefit from wearing it throughout the day.

Pay attention to how you feel. You might notice an immediate boost in energy or a gradual increase over several days. Everyone's response can be different. Drinking plenty of water can enhance the effectiveness of the patches. Hydration is key to maintaining energy levels.

Enhancing Sleep Patterns

As we age, our body's natural production of melatonin, the hormone that regulates sleep-wake cycles, decreases. Coupled with fluctuating hormone levels and increased stress, this decline can lead to difficulties in falling asleep and staying asleep. Insufficient sleep triggers a rise in cortisol, the stress hormone that further disrupts sleep cycles. The consequences are far-reaching: impaired learning ability, poor memory retention, slower metabolism, and overall hormonal imbalance.

LifeWave Silent Nights patches are designed to tackle these sleep challenges head-on by naturally boosting melatonin production without the need for outside supplements or medications[18]. By using phototherapy—a method we've discussed in previous chapters—the patches work through gentle stimulation of specific points on the body to encourage melatonin release.

Imagine waking up after a full night of restful sleep—clear-minded, energetic, and ready to take on the day. That's what users often report after incorporating Silent Nights into their nightly routine.

1. **Enhanced Quality of Sleep**: Users have experienced deeper and more restorative sleep with Silent Nights patches. Instead of light dozing or disrupted nights, the patches have allowed many to reach those essential deep sleep stages where true rest and recuperation occur.

2. **Improved Length of Sleep**: Struggling with waking up too early or tossing and turning for hours? Silent Nights helps extend total sleep time by maintaining melatonin levels throughout the night so you can enjoy longer periods of uninterrupted rest.

3. **Encouraged Natural Melatonin Production**: Unlike traditional supplements or drugs that introduce synthetic hormones into your body, Silent Nights works in harmony with your biology. This natural approach encourages your brain's own melanin release, helping alleviate disruptions without unwanted side effects.

Steps for Using Silent Nights Patches

1. Decide when you want to prepare for bed each night.
2. Place one Silent Nights patch on clean skin either on your right temple or under your right foot before sleeping.

3. Enjoy waking up refreshed without grogginess or dependency on other aids.

By making these simple steps part of your evening ritual, better snoozing becomes second nature.

While the patches are incredibly effective on their own, combining them with good sleep hygiene practices magnifies their effectiveness tremendously. Keeping a regular bed schedule, indulging in calming pre-sleep rituals such as reading or meditating, maintaining a cool bedroom environment—all these rich practices alongside using Silent Nights can see you attaining the restful nights that will have friends asking your secret.

Strengthening Mental Focus

Mental focus is all about concentration—the ability to zero in on a specific task or thought without getting distracted. For those days when you need to keep your brain sharp and your thoughts clear, certain LIFEWAVE patches could be the supportive companion you're looking for. We're talking specifically about the Y-Age Aeon Patch, Y-Age Glutathione, and Y-age Carnosine. Let's explore how these can potentially give your mental faculties a helpful nudge.

Y-Age Aeon Patch

The Y-Age Aeon patch is designed to help reduce stress and inflammation. Stress can be a BIG roadblock to mental focus; when we're stressed, our brains can feel overwhelmed, making it hard to concentrate. The Aeon patch helps by promoting a sense of calmness and well-being.

1. **Boosts Mental Clarity:** By reducing stress, the Aeon patch allows your mind to clear up and regain focus, making it easier to tackle tasks and stay productive.
2. **Lowers Inflammation:** Chronic inflammation has been linked to brain fog. By addressing inflammation, this patch helps keep your brain sharp.

Y-Age Glutathione Patch

Glutathione is often called the *"master antioxidant"* because of its ability to neutralize free radicals and reduce oxidative stress in the body.

1. **Enhances Detoxification:** A healthy brain is a clear brain. The Glutathione patch supports your body's natural detox processes, which can help improve mental clarity.

2. **Supports Neurotransmitter Function:** Glutathione helps in the function of neurotransmitters, the brain's chemical messengers. By improving neurotransmitter balance, this patch can help enhance your mood and focus.

Y-Age Carnosine Patch

Finally, we have the Y-Age Carnosine patch. Carnosine is a powerful peptide that has gained attention for its potential benefits in brain health.

1. **Protects Against Cognitive Decline:** Carnosine has neuroprotective properties, which means it can help preserve brain health as we age. This translates to better focus and memory retention.

2. **Improves Energy Levels:** When your energy levels are up, your ability to concentrate often follows suit. The Carnosine patch supports overall vitality, which can make a big difference in your daily focus.

PAIN TYPE	KEY BENEFITS	FOCUS ENHANCEMENT
Y-Age Aeon	Reduces stress, lowers inflammation	Boosts mental clarity
Y-Age Glutathione	Enhances detoxification, supports neurotransmitter function	Improves mood and focus
Y-Age Carnosine	Protects against cognitive decline, improves energy levels	Increases concentration

Using these patches is simple. Just stick one patch on a clean, dry area of your skin, like your arm or shoulder. You can wear it for up to 12 hours a day. Many people choose to use them during times when they need extra focus, like during work hours or while studying.

Supporting Immune Function

Our immune system is like our body's defense line against viruses, bacteria, and other harmful invaders. When it's working well, you're more likely to fight off colds, flu, and other illnesses with ease. On the flip side, a weakened immune system can leave you feeling run down and more susceptible to getting sick.

The LifeWave X39 and AEON patches are designed to enhance your body's natural healing processes, and they can specifically support immune function. Let's break down how each patch contributes to this goal.

X39 Patch

The X39 designed to stimulate your body to produce more of its own peptides, which are critical for cellular repair and regeneration. One important peptide that X39 helps boost is called GHK-Cu. Research has shown that this peptide plays a significant role in immune regulation. Besides that, X39 also supports overall vitality and energy, which is vital when your body is fighting off illness.

Here are a few key benefits of using the X39 patch for immune function:

1. **Increased Energy Levels:** When you have more energy, your body can better fight off infections.
2. **Enhanced Cellular Repair:** This means faster recovery from illness or injury.
3. **Improved Overall Well-being:** Feeling good physically often translates into feeling well emotionally too, which can help in fighting off sickness.

AEON Patch

This patch is all about reducing stress and promoting a balanced state in your body. Stress can significantly impact your immune system—when you're stressed, your body releases cortisol, which can suppress immune function. By using the AEON patch, you're helping to manage stress, which in turn supports your immune system.

Here are the main benefits of the AEON patch for immune support:

1. **Stress Reduction:** Less stress means a stronger immune response.

2. **Improved Sleep Quality:** Good sleep is essential for a well-functioning immune system.

3. **Balanced Mood:** Feeling good mentally can contribute to better physical health.

Now that you know the benefits, let's talk about how to use these patches effectively. Here's a simple guideline:

PAIN TYPE	HOW TO USE	FREQUENCY
X39	Apply to a clean area on the body (like the back of the neck)	Wear for 12 hours a day, then take a break for 12 hours.
AEON	Place on the body's acupuncture points (like the inner wrist)	Wear continuously for best results.

Feel free to rotate where you place the patches, as long as they're clean and dry. Also, remember to listen to your body. Some people may feel immediate relief, while others might take a little longer to notice changes.

BOOK 5

Real-Life Applications

Personal Transformation Case Studies

Imagine plugging into untapped energy resources within your body or easing those aches and pains without drugs or complex treatments. People across the globe have experienced significant personal transformations thanks to LifeWave patches, and here are a few inspiring examples.

Overcoming Fatigue

Like many of us, Lisa led a busy life. Between work, family obligations, and trying to squeeze in some personal time, she found herself constantly drained. No matter how much she tried to rest, that nagging fatigue wouldn't budge. She felt like she was running on empty.

After hearing about LifeWave patches from a friend, Lisa decided to give them a try. She started with the *Energy Enhancer* patches, which are designed to boost energy levels and combat fatigue. The first night, she placed the patches on her body as instructed and went to sleep.

To her surprise, when Lisa woke up the next morning, she felt different. Instead of the usual sluggishness, she noticed a noticeable increase in her energy. Encouraged, she continued using the patches daily. Over the next few weeks, Lisa found herself not only more energized but also more productive. She could focus better at work, play actively with her kids, and even take on new hobbies she had long neglected.

ASPECT	BEFORE LIFEWAVE PATCHES	AFTER LIFEWAVE PATCHES
Energy Levels	Low	High
Work Productivity	Struggling	Improved
Family Engagement	Limited	Active
Personal Hobbies	Neglected	Rediscovered

Lisa's experience shows how introducing LifeWave patches can completely revitalize your energy levels, which can be a game-changer in your daily life.

Enhancing Mood and Well-Being

Emily had always been the life of the party, but over the last year, she noticed her mood took a downturn. Life's stresses were beginning to weigh her down, affecting her motivation and overall outlook. She wanted to feel like herself again but was unsure where to start.

After some research, Emily learned about the Y-Age patches, which are intended to support mood and emotional balance. Feeling hopeful, she decided to incorporate them into her daily routine. She placed the patches on specific points as recommended and committed to using them consistently.

Within a week, Emily noticed subtle changes. She felt more stable in her emotions and found herself smiling more often. Social events that once seemed overwhelming became enjoyable again. She felt lighter and more engaged in conversations, which reignited her sense of connection with friends and family.

ASPECT	BEFORE LIFEWAVE PATCHES	AFTER LIFEWAVE PATCHES
Emotional Stability	Fluctuating	Balanced
Social Engagement	Withdrawn	Reconnected
Motivation	Low	High
Overall Well-Being	Diminished	Enhanced

Emily's journey illustrates how the right tools, like LifeWave patches, can help you regain balance in your mood and enhance your overall well-being.

Both Lisa and Emily have found personal transformations through their experiences with LifeWave patches. If you're looking for a change or want to enhance your daily experience, consider giving LifeWave patches a try. You might just discover the transformation you've been longing for.

Clinical Evidence

Clinical studies have explored various aspects of how these patches work, and the results can help you understand their potential benefits. In a double-blind, placebo-controlled trial, participants were divided into two groups—one group used the patches, while the other group received a placebo. The researchers measured pain levels before, during, and after the use of the patches. The findings showed that individuals using LifeWave patches reported a big reduction in pain compared to those using the placebo[19].

STUDY FOCUS	RESULTS
Pain Relief	70% of participants using patches reported relief within 30 minutes.
Sleep Quality	65% reported improved sleep quality after consistent use.
Stress Reduction	Participants noted a 40% decrease in stress levels over a month.

Many people struggle with getting a good night's rest, and the LifeWave patches might be a helpful tool. In a study focusing on sleep quality, participants who used the patches over a four-week period noted improvements in their sleep duration and quality. They also reported feeling more energized during the day. It's pretty impressive when you think about how something as simple as a patch can have such a positive impact on your sleep!

Stress, another common issue, was also evaluated in some studies. Participants using the LifeWave patches reported feeling calmer and less anxious. The clinical evidence suggested that these patches could help lower stress levels, making it easier for individuals to manage their daily lives.

Additional Research Highlights:

1. **Healthy Aging**: Some studies indicated that LifeWave patches could support healthy aging by promoting cellular function and energy levels. Participants in these studies experienced an increase in overall vitality and a reduction in feelings of fatigue.

2. **Improved Circulation:** Another area of research looked at the impact of the patches on circulation. Improved blood flow can lead to better oxygen and nutrient delivery throughout the body. Participants noted significant improvements in their circulation and overall comfort.

It's essential to emphasize that while the evidence is promising, individual results may vary. What works wonders for one person might not have the same effect on another. This is why it's important to listen to your body and monitor how you feel when using the patches.

One of the great things about LifeWave patches is that they are generally considered safe. Most users experience no adverse effects, but it's always good to consult with a healthcare professional if you have specific concerns or conditions. Using the patches is super simple—just apply them to clean, dry skin, and you're good to go!

Athlete Testimonials

When it comes to enhancing performance and recovery, athletes are always on the lookout for ways to gain an edge. One product that has gained significant attention in the athletic community is LifeWave patches. These patches have been reported to help with everything from pain relief to improved endurance.

One name that stands out is the legendary Mike Tyson. Famous for his boxing prowess, Tyson has openly shared how LifeWave patches have helps his recovery and performance. In interviews, he has mentioned that as a professional athlete, he's faced his share of injuries and fatigue. The rigorous training and competition often left him feeling worn out. After discovering LifeWave patches, he found a way to enhance his recovery time. Tyson reported feeling more energized and focused during his training sessions. He said that the patches seemed to aid in reducing soreness and speeding up his healing process, allowing him to train harder and push his limits while maintaining peak performance[20].

But he's not the only one—many athletes have found great benefits from these innovative patches. Let's look real stories and testimonials from athletes who have tried LifeWave patches, along with the results they've experienced.

1. **Sarah Johnson – Professional Runner**: Sarah, a professional marathon runner, turned to LifeWave patches after suffering from chronic shin splints. She reports that using the patches during her training significantly reduced her pain levels and accelerated her recovery time.

"I was amazed at how quickly I bounced back from long runs. The patches have been a game-changer for me!"

2. **David Lee – MMA Fighter**: David has been in the MMA circuit for years and often deals with the wear and tear of training. He started using LifeWave patches to help alleviate soreness after intense fight camps.

"I can honestly say these patches have helped me stay in the game longer. Recovery is key in my sport, and LifeWave has made a noticeable difference."

3. **Jessica Tran – CrossFit Champion**: Jessica was skeptical at first but decided to give LifeWave patches a try after hearing about them from fellow athletes. She found they helped her manage muscle fatigue and enhanced her performance during competitions.

"I noticed I could push myself harder in workouts without feeling the usual fatigue. I'm definitely sticking with these!"

The testimonials from athletes using LifeWave patches are overwhelmingly positive. Whether it's enhanced performance, quicker recovery, increased energy, or better mental clarity, these patches seem to offer practical benefits for those in the athletic community. Remember, everyone's experience is unique, and it's always a good idea to listen to your body and consult with a healthcare professional if you're considering trying them out.

Measuring Outcomes

You might be wondering, *"How do I know if these patches are actually working for me"* When it comes to using LifeWave patches, one of the best things you can do is keep track of your experiences. This isn't just about enjoying the moment; it's about gathering valuable data that you can refer back to. So, let's dive into how you can measure your outcomes effectively.

1. **Define Your Goals**: Before you even put on a patch, take a moment to think about what you want to achieve. Are you looking to relieve pain, boost your energy, improve sleep, or enhance overall wellness? Having clear goals will help you measure your outcomes more effectively. Write these down so you can refer back to them later. Here's a simple table to help you get started:

GOAL	DESIRED OUTCOME
Pain Relief	Reduction in pain level
Increased Energy	Feeling more energetic throughout the day

Improved Sleep Quality	Falling asleep faster and better rest
Enhanced Recovery	Reduced recovery time after activity

2. **Keep a Journal**: This might sound a bit old-school, but keeping a journal is one of the best ways to track how you're feeling. Make a habit of jotting down your daily experiences with the patches. Note the date, the specific patch you used, and any sensations or changes you felt throughout the day. You can even rate your experiences on a scale of 1 to 10. Here's a simple format you can use:

DATE	PATCH USED	DAILY RATING (1-10)	NOTES
MM/DD/YYYY	Energy Patch	7	Felt more energetic in the afternoon
MM/DD/YYYY	Sleep Patch	8	Fell asleep faster than usual
MM/DD/YYYY	Pain Relief Patch	5	Pain level decreased significantly

3. **Track Physical Symptoms**: If you're using LifeWave patches for specific health issues, it's important to monitor your physical symptoms closely. This may include pain levels, sleep quality, or any other symptoms related to your goals. You can use a simple chart to note changes:

SYMPTOM	BEFORE USING PATCHES	AFTER ONE WEEK	AFTER ONE MONTH
Pain Level	8/10	5/10	3/10
Energy Level	4/10	6/10	8/10
Sleep Quality	5/10	7/10	9/10

4. **Reflect on Your Experience**: After a month or so of using the patches, take a moment to reflect on your overall experience. Look back through your journal to see patterns. Are you feeling better? Are your symptoms improving? Comparing your notes will help you see the bigger picture.

5. **Consider Talking with Others**: Sometimes, it can be really helpful to speak with others who are also using LifeWave patches. Join online forums or local groups to share experiences and tips. You may discover new ways to measure outcomes or find support from people on similar journeys.

To see the best results from LifeWave patches, use them regularly as directed. Measuring your outcomes will only be effective if you stick to the routine. Take a moment to remind yourself of your goals, and don't hesitate to make adjustments based on your findings.

If you're unsure about how to track your outcomes or if you want a deeper analysis, consider consulting with a healthcare professional familiar with LifeWave patches. They can help guide you in measuring your progress effectively.

Everyday Health Improvements

Everyday health IS not just about avoiding sickness; it's about feeling vibrant and energetic. This includes getting enough sleep, managing stress, staying active, and eating well. Each of these elements are important, and the Lifewave patches can enhance these areas seamlessly.

You need to know your health goals. Are you looking to boost your energy levels? Improve your sleep? Manage stress? Having a clear idea of what you want to achieve will guide how you use Lifewave patches effectively.

1. **Start Your Day Right**: Mornings can be rough, but they set the tone for the rest of your day. Instead of reaching for caffeine first thing, why not start with a Lifewave patch? Many users report feeling more energetic and focused when they apply a patch as part of their morning routine.

TIP: Try placing a patch on a non-sensitive area of your body, like your shoulder or wrist, after you wake up. This can help boost your energy levels and get you ready for the day.

2. **Manage Stress Throughout the Day**: Life can throw a lot at us, and sometimes it can feel overwhelming. Anxiety and stress can easily sneak into your day, but Lifewave patches can help manage those feelings. For instance, if you're heading into a stressful meeting or presentation, consider using a calming patch beforehand.

PATCH TYPE	BEST USE	TIME OF DAY
Energy Patch	To boost energy and focus	Morning
Calming Patch	To ease anxiety	Before stressful events
Sleep Patch	To help wind down	Evening

3. **Stay Active**: If you're someone who enjoys working out or staying active, Lifewave patches can be a great addition to your routine. Applying a patch before your workouts can help improve your performance and reduce fatigue. After your workout, consider using a recovery patch to ease soreness and help your muscles recover faster.

TIP: Experiment with different patches to see which ones work best for your body. Some people find they have better endurance with an energy patch, while others prefer the recovery patch post-workout.

4. **Nighttime Relaxation**: After a long day, it's important to unwind and prepare for a good night's sleep. Using a Lifewave patch designed for sleep can help you relax. Many users find that they fall asleep faster and wake up feeling more refreshed.

   a) *Dinner:* Keep it light and nutritious to avoid feeling sluggish.
   b) *Patch Application:* Apply the sleep patch about 30 minutes before bedtime.
   c) *Wind Down:* Engage in calming activities like reading or gentle stretching.

While this may not seem directly related to Lifewave patches, staying hydrated is important for overall health. Water helps your body function properly and can enhance the effectiveness of the patches. Aim for at least 8 glasses of water a day to keep your body energized and functioning at its best.

Not every patch will work the same for everyone, and that's okay! Pay attention to how your body feels and don't be afraid to mix and match. If you feel particularly stressed one day, use a calming patch; if you've had a tough workout, reach for something that promotes recovery.

Consider keeping a journal of how you feel with different patches and routines. Write down what you used, how you felt before and after, and any other observations. This can help you pinpoint what works best for you and make adjustments for even better results.

By incorporating Lifewave patches into your routine, you can tackle stress, boost energy, enhance your workouts, and improve your sleep—all in a way that feels natural. Just remember to listen to your body and adjust as needed.

BOOK 6

Overcoming Hurdles

Addressing Doubts

Let's acknowledge that doubt is a part of human nature. Whether you're trying to lose weight, learn a new skill, or use Lifewave patches, it's common to question if you're on the right track. You might be wondering if these patches will really work for you, or if you're just wasting your time and money. You're not alone; many people experience these feelings when venturing into new wellness routines.

Doubts often come from a place of uncertainty. Maybe you've heard mixed reviews from friends or seen some skeptical comments online. It's okay to wonder whether Lifewave patches can truly deliver results. To tackle these doubts effectively, let's break down some of the most common questions that pop into people's minds:

1. Do Lifewave Patches Really Work?

The Lifewave patches are designed using specific technologies that aim to promote wellness. While individual experiences may vary, many users report positive outcomes, such as increased energy, improved sleep, and better overall health. Research and testimonials can help you make sense of the benefits. If you're still skeptical, consider reaching out to thriving communities online. Individuals often share their personal success stories, which can be quite encouraging.

2. Will They Work for Me?

This question often leads to some self-doubt. Understand that everyone's body is unique, and what works for one person may not work the same way for another. However, it's essential to remember that many users have found a positive impact with consistent use of Lifewave patches. Give yourself the grace to experiment. Maybe commit to using the patches for a specific period, like 30 days, and keep track of how you feel. You could be pleasantly surprised!

3. Are There Any Side Effects or Risks?

Like any wellness product, it's wise to be informed. The Lifewave patches are generally considered safe, as they are non-invasive and made from materials that are skin-friendly. However, if you have any specific health concerns, it's best to consult with a healthcare professional before starting. They can help you understand if the patches are a good fit for you.

One practical way to ease your doubts is by keeping a record of your experiences. This could be a chart where you jot down:

DATE	PATCH USED	DURATION OF USE	SYMPTOMS/ FEELINGS	NOTES
01/01/2025	Energy	8 hours	Felt energized	Great start to the day
01/02/2025	Sleep	8 hours	Slept well	Woke up refreshed
01/03/2025	Pain Relief	6 hours	Pain decreased	Happy with results

By documenting your journey, you create a reference point that not only gives you insights into what works but also helps combat doubts. When you look back and see your own progress, it can provide motivation and confidence.

Sometimes, the best way to overcome doubts is through connection. Engage with communities of Lifewave users on social media or forums. Sharing your concerns and hearing from others who've encountered similar doubts can be incredibly reassuring. Plus, you might pick up tips and tricks along the way!

Resolving Improper Use

Improper use of Lifewave patches can be a hurdle, but it's one that's easily overcome with a little attention and care. By following the guidelines for proper use and being mindful of your body's responses, you can maximize the benefits of these patches. Let's go through some tips to help you get it right and enjoy the full benefits of these amazing patches.

1. **Placement of the Patches:** Each patch has specific points where it works best. If you're using a patch for pain relief, for instance, you'll want to place it directly over the area that hurts. If you're not sure where to put it, refer to the instructions that come with the patches or check the LifeWave website for detailed guidance.

2. **Not Following Instructions**: We know that reading instructions can be a drag, but it's important when using LifeWave patches. Each type of patch comes with specific guidelines for usage, including duration and frequency. Ignoring these instructions might mean you're not getting the full benefits.

Make sure to take a few moments to read through the material that comes with your patches, or check online for videos and guides. Following the instructions helps you avoid unnecessary frustration and ensures you're using the patches effectively.

3. **Using Multiple Patches Incorrectly**: Sometimes, people think that using multiple patches at once will boost the effects. While there are combination patches that work well together, using too many or the wrong types at the same time can lead to less effective results. It's best to stick to the recommendations provided by LifeWave.

If you're curious about combining patches, reach out to customer support or consult with a practitioner who's knowledgeable about LifeWave products. They can give you insights into what works best together.

4. **Skin Preparation**: Did you know that how you prepare your skin can impact how well the patches stick and work? Before applying a patch, make sure your skin is clean and dry. Avoid using lotions, oils, or other products on the area where you'll place the patch; this can create a barrier that prevents it from adhering properly.

If you're concerned about skin irritation, consider testing the patch on a small area first. If you experience any redness or discomfort, stop using it and consult with a healthcare professional.

5. **Monitoring Your Body's Response**: After you apply a patch, pay attention to how your body responds. If you notice any unusual symptoms or side effects, it's best to remove the patch and give your body a break. LifeWave patches should not cause significant discomfort; if they do, that's a sign something is off.

Again, keep a journal of how you feel after using the patches. Documenting your experiences can help you identify what works best for you and what doesn't.

6. **Checking Expiration Dates**: It may sound silly, but make sure your patches are still good to use! Patches can lose their effectiveness over time, so always check the expiration date on the packaging. Using expired patches may lead to less effective results, and we don't want that!

Remember, overcoming the hurdle of improper use takes time and patience. The more you learn about how to use LifeWave patches correctly, the better your experience will be. Follow these tips, stay informed, and don't hesitate to reach out for help if you need it.

Breaking Plateaus

Plateau is that moment when you feel like you're not moving forward despite your efforts. In Lifewave patches, this might mean you're not seeing the results you'd hoped for after a few weeks or months of use. It's normal! Almost everyone experiences plateaus at some point, whether it's with fitness, weight loss, or even health improvement using patches.

Assess Your Current Routine

Assess what you're currently doing. Take a moment to jot down how you're using your Lifewave patches. Here's a table to help you track your patch usage:

DAY	PATCH USED	DURATION (HOURS)	NOTES/FEELINGS
MON	Patch 1	12	Felt energized
TUE	Patch 1	12	No change
WED	Patch 2	8	Minor headache
THU	Patch 2	8	Good sleep
FRI	Patch 3	10	Felt tired
SAT	Patch 1	12	No noticeable change
SUN	Patch 3	12	Felt great!

This table will help you identify patterns in your usage. Are you using the patches consistently? Are you rotating different patches as recommended? Sometimes, simply increasing the duration or changing the patches can yield better results.

Consider Your Environment

Your environment can also impact how effective the patches are. Factors such as stress, diet, sleep quality, and physical activity play a huge role in how your body responds to the patches. Consider the following:

1. **Stress Levels:** Are you feeling more stressed than usual? Stress can hinder your body's ability to heal and adapt.

2. **Diet and Hydration:** Are you eating balanced meals and staying hydrated? Dehydration can lead to fatigue and headaches, which might mask the benefits of the patches.

3. **Sleep Quality:** Are you getting enough rest? Sleep is crucial for recovery and health maintenance.

Take some time to reflect on these aspects of your life, and make any necessary adjustments. Small changes can lead to big results.

Experiment with Your Patch Routine

If you're feeling stuck, it might be time to shake things up a bit. Here are a few tips:

1. **Change Your Patch Placement:** Sometimes, simply moving the patches to a different spot on your body can make a difference in how they work for you.

2. **Try Different Patches:** If you've been using the same patch for a while, consider trying a different one to see if you notice any changes. Each patch has its unique benefits, and mixing things up might help you break through that plateau.

3. **Adjust Timing:** Experiment with the time of day you apply your patches. Some people find that using patches at night works better for them, while others might benefit from daytime application.

Another way to overcome plateaus is to connect with others who are on the same journey. Online forums, social media groups, or in-person meetups can provide valuable insights. You might discover new tips or tricks that others have found helpful.

Keep track of your changes! Use a journal or an app to record how you feel and any adjustments you make. This ongoing record will help you see patterns over time and understand what works best for you.

Managing Initial Discomfort

It's important to understand that experiencing some discomfort when starting any new health regimen is quite normal. Your body is adjusting to new stimuli, and with Lifewave patches, it's no different. Many users report varying levels of discomfort, and while it can be annoying, it usually doesn't last long.

DISCOMFORT	DESCRIPTION	DURATION	WHAT TO DO
Light Headache	A mild headache that can occur as your body adjusts.	1-3 days	Stay hydrated, rest, and consider reducing caffeine.
Fatigue	Feeling a bit more tired than usual.	1-2 days	Ensure you're getting enough sleep and take short naps if needed.
Soreness	Some users report slight soreness where the patch is applied.	1-2 days	Change the patch location, and make sure to apply it to clean, dry skin.
Skin Irritation	This can happen if the skin is sensitive.	Varies	Remove the patch and allow your skin to breathe. Use a sensitive skin patch if needed.

Tips for Managing Discomfort

1. Drinking plenty of water helps your body detox and can alleviate some discomfort. Aim for at least eight glasses a day, or more if you're active.

2. Your body may need a little extra downtime to adjust. Don't hesitate to take it easy if you feel fatigued. Listen to your body; it knows what it needs.

3. If you're feeling soreness or irritation where the patch is applied, try rotating the area. This can help prevent sensitivity. Aim for different spots on your body, like your arms, legs, or back.

4. Keep track of any discomfort you experience along with the date and patch usage. This information can be helpful if you need to adjust your routine later.

5. Join online forums or local groups of Lifewave users. They can provide support and share their experiences. Sometimes, just knowing you aren't alone can be comforting.

If discomfort persists beyond a few days or worsens, it's a good idea to consult a healthcare professional. There are many factors at play when using patches, and it's always better to be safe.

While dealing with initial discomfort can be frustrating, keeping your end goals in mind can help. Many users report feeling significantly better once their body adjusts. The patches are designed to support your overall wellbeing, so hang in there! The discomfort is often temporary, and the benefits can be life-changing.

BOOK 7
Lifestyle and Results

Diet and Exercise Synergies

Your diet consists of the foods you eat, which deliver the necessary nutrients your body needs to function properly. Exercise, on the other hand, refers to the physical activities you engage in to strengthen your body, improve your cardiovascular health, and boost your mood.

When you pair a healthy diet with regular exercise, you're not just improving one aspect of your health; you're amplifying the benefits of both. Together, they can enhance your energy levels, improve your mood, and even aid in better sleep—all crucial for anyone looking to maintain or improve their health.

The Power of a Balanced Diet

So, what does a balanced diet look like? Here's a breakdown of essential food groups you should aim for:

FOOD GROUP	EXAMPLES	BENEFITS
Fruits & Vegetables	Apples, leafy greens, berries	Packed with vitamins, minerals, and antioxidants; they support your immune system and overall health. Aim for a variety of colors on your plate!
Lean Proteins	Chicken, turkey, fish, beans, legumes	Essential for muscle repair and growth. Protein helps keep you satiated and supports recovery after exercise.
Whole Grains	Brown rice, quinoa, oats	Provide energy and help maintain stable blood sugar levels. They're also rich in fiber, which is great for digestion.
Healthy Fats	Avocado, olive oil, nuts, seeds	Incorporate sources like avocados, nuts, seeds, and olive oil. They help with nutrient absorption and provide long-lasting energy.

Aim to fill half your plate with fruits and vegetables, a quarter with lean protein, and a quarter with whole grains. This balance can help you feel full and satisfied while providing the nutrients your body craves. Don't forget to drink plenty of water! Staying hydrated is important for your overall health and can highly impact your energy levels and exercise performance.

When you fuel your body with the right foods, you'll likely notice that your workouts feel easier and more effective. You'll have more energy, recover faster, and even feel better mentally.

How Exercise Complements Your Diet

Regular physical activity does wonders for your body. It helps with weight management, boosts your immune system, and increases your mood through the release of endorphins—the *"feel-good"* hormones. Different types of exercise can have varying effects on your body:

1. **Cardiovascular Exercise:** Activities like running, cycling, or even brisk walking increase your heart rate and improve blood circulation. This is essential for overall health and supports metabolism, helping to burn off those extra calories from your meals.

2. **Strength Training:** Lifting weights or doing body-weight exercises like push-ups and squats builds muscle. The more muscle you have, the higher your resting metabolic rate, meaning you'll burn more calories even when you're not exercising.

3. **Flexibility and Balance:** Yoga and stretching not only improve flexibility but also help with muscle recovery and stress reduction, which can significantly complement your diet choices.

It's important to find a balance. For example, if you focus only on cardio, you might not be building enough muscle. On the flip side, if you only lift weights without incorporating cardio, you might miss out on important heart health benefits.

Creating a Balanced Routine

To get the best results, aim for a balanced routine that includes both a well-rounded diet and a mix of exercise types. Here's a weekly plan you can follow:

DAY	EXERCISE TYPE	MEAL FOCUS
MON	Cardio (30 mins)	Lean proteins and veggies
TUE	Strength training	Whole grains and healthy fats
WED	Flexibility/Yoga	Fruits and hydration
THU	Cardio (30 mins)	Balanced meals with protein
FRI	Strength training	Nutrient-dense snacks
SAT	Active Recovery (walk)	High-fiber meals
SUN	Rest day	Meal prep for the week

The key to making the most out of your diet and exercise routine is consistency. It's not about being perfect every single day, but rather making small, sustainable changes that you can stick to in the long run.

1. Dedicate a day to prepare healthy meals and snacks for the week. This helps you avoid unhealthy choices when you're busy or tired.
2. Don't forget about water! It's essential for digestion and can also help you feel full, reducing unnecessary snacking.
3. Pay attention to how your body feels. If you're tired or sore, don't hesitate to adjust your workout plan or give yourself a break. Recovery is just as important as the workouts themselves.
4. Focus on achievable targets, whether it's drinking more water, eating more vegetables, or gradually increasing your workout duration. Celebrate your wins, no matter how small!

Incorporating a balanced diet with regular exercise can lead to optimal health outcomes. Remember, it's about the lifestyle changes you make, not just quick fixes. So, take it one step at a time, and enjoy the journey to a healthier you!

Daily Routines with Patches

Planning a daily routine when using these patches is like following a fitness routine to achieve better health. You want your body to adapt to a pattern so it can respond optimally to the patches. Now that you're familiar with the LifeWave patches and their incredible benefits, let's discuss how you can incorporate them into your daily routine for the best results. It's all about consistency and knowing when and how to use them.

Morning Routine

1. **Start Your Day Right**: As soon as you wake up, take a moment to set your intentions for the day. Think about what you want to achieve, whether it's increased energy or reduced stress.

2. **Apply Your Patches**: Place the patches on clean and dry skin in the morning. The best spots are usually on the upper body, like the back of your neck or your shoulder. If you're using patches for energy, try placing them on your wrists or behind your ears.

TIP: For best results, you can apply a patch like the Energy Enhancer patch before breakfast. It helps boost your energy levels right from the start!

3. **Stay Hydrated**: Drink a glass of water after applying your patches. Staying hydrated is key to maximizing the benefits of the patches, as water helps your body function optimally.

Midday Check-In

1. **Monitor Your Energy Levels**: Around midday, take a moment to check in with yourself. Are you feeling energized? If not, consider adding a second Energy Enhancer patch or a patch that suits your needs, like the Ice Wave for any discomfort.

2. **Snack Smart**: Pair your patches with healthy snacks. Nuts, fruits, or yogurt can keep your energy up and your body fueled.

3. **Reapply as Needed**: If you're using a patch for specific pain relief or stress management, consider reapplying after about 12 hours. Just remember: don't apply multiple patches in the same spot. Give your skin a break by moving them to a different area.

Evening Wind Down

1. **Reflect on Your Day**: As your day winds down, think about how your patches influenced your day. Did you feel more energetic, less stressed, or did you notice any changes in discomfort? This reflection will help you understand which patches worked best for you.

2. **Prepare for Sleep**: If you're using patches for relaxation or sleep, like the Silent Nights patch, apply it about 30 minutes before bedtime. Place it on your wrist or the back of your neck to promote a restful night.

3. **Create a Relaxing Environment**: Turn off screens, dim the lights, and perhaps do some light stretching or meditation while the patch works its magic. This will enhance the calming effects of the patches and help you unwind.

Weekly Routine

1. **Patch Rotation**: Consider rotating the patches throughout the week. For example, if you're using the Energy Enhancer patch in the morning, you can switch to the Ice Wave for pain

management later in the week. This prevents your body from becoming too accustomed to one patch.

2. **Evaluate and Adjust**: At the end of the week, take some time to assess how the patches have affected your overall well-being. Keep a journal or notes to track your energy levels, stress, and any discomfort. This will help you make informed choices going forward.

TIME OF DAY	ACTION	PATCH RECOMMENDATION
Morning	Apply patches on clean skin	Energy Enhancer
Midday	Check in on energy, reapply if needed	Ice Wave (if needed)
Evening	Reflect, relax, and prepare for sleep	Silent Nights
Weekly	Rotate patches and evaluate results	Varies based on need

Following this type of structured routine helps establish consistency and enhances effectiveness across different patches from LifeWave's lineup. Tracking changes in how you feel over weeks or months helps you make informed decisions about when to switch things up or keep them going strong.

Importance of Hydration

Proper hydration is important for our bodies to function well, particularly when we're using techniques like the LifeWave patches. Our bodies are made up of about 60% water. It's a vital component for almost every process in our bodies, from regulating temperature to transporting nutrients. When we're not adequately hydrated, we can experience fatigue, headaches, and even decreased concentration. Staying hydrated helps keep our energy levels up, supports digestion, and helps our skin look its best.

Here are some specific benefits of staying hydrated, especially when you're looking to enhance your wellness journey:

1. **Boosts Energy Levels:** Dehydration can lead to feelings of fatigue. By drinking enough water, you're helping your body produce energy more efficiently.
2. **Enhances Mood:** Studies show that even mild dehydration can affect your mood and lead to feelings of anxiety and irritability. Staying hydrated can help keep your spirits up.

3. **Aids Digestion:** Water is essential for digestion. It helps break down food so your body can absorb nutrients. Plus, it prevents constipation.

4. **Improves Physical Performance:** If you're exercising or using patches to enhance recovery, hydration is key. Dehydration can lead to decreased performance, muscle cramps, and longer recovery times.

5. **Supports Skin Health:** Drinking enough water keeps your skin hydrated and can help reduce the appearance of fine lines and dryness.

6. **Flushes Out Toxins:** Water helps your kidneys filter waste from the blood and expel it through urine. Staying hydrated supports this natural detox process.

While the "8 glasses a day" rule is popular, individual water needs can vary based on factors like age, weight, activity level, and climate.

FACTOR	SUGGESTED DAILY INTAKE
Average Adult	2.7 to 3.7 liters (91 to 125 oz)
Active Individuals	3.7 to 4.5 liters (125 to 152 oz)
Hot Weather	Increase by 1 to 2 liters (34 to 68 oz)
Pregnant Women	3.0 liters (101 oz)
Breastfeeding Women	3.8 liters (128 oz)

These amounts include all fluids consumed, not just water. Remember that foods like fruits and vegetables also contribute to hydration.

Tips to Stay Hydrated

1. Always have a water bottle with you. Having it on hand makes it easier to sip throughout the day.

2. : Use your phone or an app to remind you to drink water regularly. It's easy to forget when you're busy!

3. If plain water doesn't excite you, try adding lemon, cucumber, or mint for a flavor boost.

4. Incorporate foods like watermelon, cucumbers, oranges, and strawberries into your diet. They are delicious and hydrating!

5. A simple way to check hydration is by looking at the color of your urine. Light yellow usually indicates good hydration, while dark yellow suggests you should drink more.

Long-Term Impact of Using LifeWave Patches

Many people are discovering the positive changes these patches can bring to their lives. These patches are designed to stimulate the body's natural healing abilities. By using specific patches, people often experience relief from various issues, including pain, stress, and fatigue. But what happens if you keep using them consistently?

Enhanced Energy Levels

One of the most commonly reported long-term benefits is increased energy levels. Many users find that after several weeks of consistent patch use, they feel more energized and less fatigued throughout the day. This can be especially helpful if you have a hectic schedule or are juggling multiple responsibilities. Over time, users have reported:

- ✓ Improved stamina during workouts.
- ✓ Less afternoon slumps in energy, making it easier to stay productive.
- ✓ Better quality sleep, which contributes to feeling refreshed and alert.

Pain Management

If you're someone who struggles with chronic pain, you might be pleasantly surprised by the long-term effects of using LifeWave patches. Many individuals find that their pain levels decrease significantly after regular use. This can lead to:

- ✓ Reduced reliance on over-the-counter medications for pain relief.
- ✓ Improved mobility and flexibility, allowing you to enjoy daily activities without discomfort.
- ✓ A better overall mood, as chronic pain can often lead to frustration and anxiety.

Stress Reduction

Stress is a huge part of modern life, and managing it effectively is essential for your overall health. Long-term use of LifeWave patches can promote relaxation and help alleviate feelings of stress. Users often notice:

- ✓ A greater sense of calm in stressful situations.
- ✓ Better coping mechanisms when faced with challenges.

✓ Improved relationships, as stress can impact how we interact with others.

Immune System Support

Another exciting aspect of continuous use of LifeWave patches is their potential impact on your immune system. A well-functioning immune system is vital for overall health, and many users report feeling less susceptible to common illnesses after consistent use. Over time, you might experience:

✓ Fewer colds and infections.

✓ A quicker recovery time when you do fall ill.

✓ Enhanced overall vitality, allowing you to enjoy life to the fullest.

Emotional Well-Being

Maintaining a positive emotional state is crucial for a happy life. Long-term users of LifeWave patches frequently discuss improvements in mood and emotional balance. This can lead to:

✓ Fewer mood swings and greater emotional stability.

✓ Increased motivation to pursue goals and interests.

✓ Enhanced self-esteem, as feeling better physically can contribute to a better outlook on life.

BENEFIT	SHORT-TERM EFFECTS	LONG-TERM EFFECTS
Energy Levels	Initial energy boost	Sustained energy throughout the day
Pain Management	Temporary relief	Reduced chronic pain
Stress Reduction	Immediate calm	Long-term stress management
Immune Support	Minor boost	Fewer illnesses, quicker recovery
Emotional Well-Being	Temporary mood lift	Greater emotional stability

The long-term impact of using LifeWave patches can be incredibly beneficial, touching various aspects of your health and well-being. Remember, everyone's experience will vary, and it's important to listen to your body. If you're considering incorporating LifeWave patches into your daily routine, take the plunge and see how they can transform your life over time.

Reflecting On Progress and Consistency

When we talk about progress, we're talking about those tangible improvements you experience over time as you use the patches. Everyone's body reacts differently, which is why consistent reflection on your journey is key. Some see immediate benefits, while others might experience subtler changes that accumulate over a few weeks.

Just like any health or wellness program, the results often come from regular use, not just haphazard application. The patches are designed to work synergistically with your body, and this harmony can take time to establish. So, make sure you're applying the patches as directed and incorporating them into your daily life.

Tracking Your Progress

It's easy to get caught up in the day-to-day grind and forget about how far you've come. By taking the time to reflect, you not only boost your motivation but also get a clearer picture of what's working and what might need some adjustments.

1. **Tracking Changes:** One of the best ways to notice progress is to keep a journal. Write down how you feel before you start using the patches, and then check in regularly. You could jot down things like pain levels, energy, mood, and sleep quality. This will give you a tangible way to see how much you've improved over time.

DATE	PATCH USED	SYMPTOMS BEFORE	SYMPTOMS AFTER	NOTES
MM/DD/YYYY	X Patch	Mild headache	No headache	Felt energized today.
MM/DD/YYYY	Y Patch	Fatigue	More alert	Slept better last night.
MM/DD/YYYY	Z Patch	Stiff neck	80% improved	Did yoga afterward.

By jotting down your experiences, you create a clear picture of your progress over time. You'll start to see patterns and may even discover which patches work best for you in different situations.

2. **Identifying Patterns:** When you reflect, you might start to notice patterns in your healing process. For example, you might find that certain patches work better for specific issues or that

specific times of day affect how you feel. Being aware of these patterns can help you tweak your approach for even better results.

3. **Celebrating Successes:** It's important to celebrate the small wins. Did you have a day where your pain was significantly reduced? Did you sleep better than usual? Acknowledging these successes can boost your confidence and keep you focused on your journey.

When you take a moment to look back at your entries, you might be surprised by how much you've improved. It's easy to forget the small wins, like getting better sleep or feeling more energized throughout the day. Reflection helps you celebrate those victories, no matter how small they may seem.

You might notice that certain patches work better during specific times. For example, perhaps the patches ease your tension more effectively after a long day at work than they do in the morning. Recognizing these trends allows you to adjust your patch usage for maximum benefit.

Consistency and Building Habits

Now, let's talk about building habits. Consistency isn't just about applying the patches; it also involves integrating them into your lifestyle. The more consistent you are, the easier it becomes to remember to use them. Here are a few tips to help you stay on track:

1. **Set Reminders:** Use your phone or calendar to set reminders for when to apply your patches. Making it a part of your daily routine will help make it second nature.

2. **Building Momentum:** Just like any habit, the more you do it, the easier it gets. If you consistently apply the patches as recommended, you're more likely to see ongoing improvements. Think of it as building momentum; each day you stick to your routine, you're laying the groundwork for even greater healing.

3. **Create a Ritual:** Consider making patch application a calming part of your day. Whether it's in the morning with your coffee or at night before bed, find a time that works for you.

4. **Adjusting Based on Feedback:** As you maintain consistency, you'll start to gather feedback from your body regarding how the patches are working for you. If you notice that a particular patch isn't having the desired effect, you can adjust your routine accordingly. This flexible approach is essential for long-term success.

5. **Stay Educated:** Knowledge is power. The more you learn about the benefits of the patches, the more motivated you'll be to use them regularly. Join online forums or groups where you can share experiences and tips with others.

6. **Be Patient:** Remember that healing and improvement take time. Don't get discouraged if you don't see immediate results. The cumulative effect of consistent use can lead to significant benefits over time.

As you continue to explore the benefits of Lifewave patches, remember to take the time to reflect on your progress and stay consistent. Each small step forward counts, and by keeping track of your experiences, you'll not only gain insight into your healing journey but also empower yourself to make informed decisions.

Building a Supportive Community Around Lifewave Practices

When you're on a health journey, sharing experiences and tips with others can make all the difference. A supportive community provides encouragement and motivation, which can help keep you accountable. Plus, you can learn from others' successes and challenges, gaining insights that you might not have discovered on your own. Here are some steps you can take to cultivate a vibrant community around Lifewave practices:

1. **Start Local Meetups**: Consider organizing regular meetups in your area. This could be a casual gathering at a café or at someone's home. You can share personal stories, experiences with Lifewave patches, and tips for better usage. This informal setting creates an inviting space for discussion and connection.

2. **Join Online Groups**: There are plenty of online forums and social media groups focused on Lifewave practices. Joining these platforms can connect you with people from all over who share your interests. Engage with posts, ask questions, and share your own experiences. Facebook groups, Instagram hashtags, and even dedicated Lifewave forums can be valuable resources.

3. **Host Webinars or Workshops**: If you're comfortable, consider hosting a webinar or workshop. This can be an excellent way to educate others about Lifewave practices and share

what you've learned. These events can be interactive, allowing participants to ask questions and share their experiences in real-time.

4. **Create a Newsletter**: A monthly newsletter can be a great way to keep your community informed. Include tips, success stories, and updates on the latest Lifewave products or practices. Encourage your community members to contribute their own tips or testimonials, fostering a sense of ownership and partnership.

5. **Encourage Social Media Engagement**: Use platforms like Instagram, Facebook, or TikTok to share your Lifewave journey. Post about your experiences with the patches, share photos, and invite others to join you. Encourage your friends and followers to use specific hashtags related to Lifewave. This can create a larger online community.

6. **Attend Lifewave Events**: Keep an eye out for Lifewave-sponsored events or seminars. Attending these gatherings can help you meet others who are passionate about Lifewave practices. It's a great way to network, share experiences, and learn from experts.

7. **Support Each Other**: Remember, the goal is to uplift each other. Celebrate each other's successes, whether it's pain relief, improved energy, or better sleep. Create an environment where everyone feels comfortable sharing their struggles too. Sometimes, just knowing someone else is going through a similar experience can be incredibly comforting.

8. **Share Resources**: As a community, you can gather resources, articles, and other educational materials related to Lifewave practices. Create a shared folder or a resource guide that everyone can access. This can include links to studies, videos, and articles that reinforce what you're learning together.

ACTIVITY	PLATFORM	FREQUENCY	PURPOSE
Local Meetups	In-person	Monthly	Share experiences, tips
Online Group Discussions	Facebook/Reddit	Weekly	Engage, ask questions
Webinars/Workshops	Zoom/YouTube	Quarterly	Educate and share knowledge
Newsletter	Email	Monthly	Keep members informed
Social Media Sharing	Instagram/Facebook	Daily/Weekly	Inspire and connect
Attendance at Lifewave Events	In-person	As available	Network and learn

BOOK 8

Advanced and Future Insights

Latest Research Updates

LifeWave patches are known for their ability to stimulate specific points on the body by using light. But what's been happening recently in terms of research? Well, there's been a surge in studies and trials that aim to understand these patches better and prove their effectiveness.

One of the most exciting recent developments has been in the area of pain management. Many users have reported significant relief from chronic pain conditions after using LifeWave patches. This has led researchers to carry out clinical trials to verify these claims. The results have been promising! One study showed that participants using LifeWave patches experienced a reduction in pain scores by as much as 70% compared to those who didn't use them.

A big focus area has also been on energy enhancement. Imagine feeling like you had a shot of espresso—but without any caffeine involved. A recent placebo-controlled study showed that wearing these patches consistently increased participants' vitality levels and reduced fatigue significantly compared to those wearing placebo patches. It's fascinating how these patches potentially influence our energy patterns.

Sleep improvement is another area where LifeWave patches have sparked interest. With so many people struggling to get adequate rest, any product offering better sleep is bound to garner attention. Recent research indicates that users report deeper sleep cycles and less restlessness when using specific LifeWave patches designed for this purpose.

Let's talk enhancement of athletic performance next—yes, athletes are now catching onto this trend too! Some studies examining muscle recovery times have shown positive results with LifeWave usage. Athletes reported quicker recovery post-exercise, allowing for better performance and less downtime between training sessions.

What's even more incredible is that there's ongoing research looking into how LifeWave patches may help support various body systems like our immune response or hormonal balance! While conclusive evidence is still needed, initial findings suggest beneficial outcomes, adding another layer of intrigue to these small yet powerful tools.

STUDY AREA	KEY FINDINGS
Pain Management	70% reduction in pain scores reported
Energy Enhancement	Increased vitality levels compared to placebo
Sleep Improvement	Deeper sleep cycles with less restlessness
Athletic Performance	Faster recovery times post-exercise
Potential System Support	Positive indications for immune response support

It's always important to remember that while research is promising, individual results can vary—each person's experience with LifeWave might be different based on various factors such as lifestyle, health status, etc.

New Patch Developments

If you've been following along, you know how incredible these patches can be for enhancing healing and overall wellness. Now, let's talk about what's new and what you can expect moving forward. Technology and research are ever-evolving, and LifeWave is no exception.

LifeWave has been hard at work developing new patches that cater to various needs. These patches not only aim to improve health but also enhance performance, recovery, and overall well-being. Here are some of the latest developments:

LifeWave X49™ Patch

The LifeWave X49™ patch represents a significant leap in fitness and strength enhancement, especially for individuals aged 40 to 81. A comprehensive study demonstrated that participants experienced improvements in fitness ranging from 31% to 70% over a 60-day usage period. This impressive result underscores the patch's capacity to stimulate energy production, enhance endurance, and optimize overall athletic performance.

By utilizing a patented technology that works through the body's own energy systems, the X49 patch is designed to elevate strength and stamina. Whether you are an athlete seeking to improve your performance or someone looking to regain vitality in your daily activities, the X49 patch offers a non-invasive and drug-free solution. Imagine being able to engage fully in your favorite activities, feeling invigorated and strong, regardless of age. This patch facilitates not just an improvement in physical capabilities, but also a renewed sense of confidence and empowerment.

Alavida Patch

The Alavida patch introduces an exciting dimension to skincare and overall health. Engineered to capture and reflect the body's infrared energy, this patch stimulates specific points on the skin, promoting cellular renewal and vitality. Users often report enhancements in their skin's appearance, citing improvements such as increased hydration and reduction in the visibility of fine lines.

The Alavida patch is particularly noteworthy for those seeking a holistic approach to skincare. By addressing skin health from within, it aligns with the principles of natural wellness, allowing for rejuvenation that transcends mere surface treatments. Moreover, the patch's ability to promote a general state of health means that it can contribute to overall well-being, fostering a sense of balance and tranquility that is essential in today's fast-paced world.

Aeon Patch

Inflammation is a root cause of many chronic conditions, making the Aeon patch an invaluable tool in the wellness arsenal. Clinically tested, this patch has been shown to effectively reduce inflammation, providing relief for individuals suffering from inflammatory pain. The ability to pair the Aeon patch with LifeWave's IceWave patches enhances its efficacy, allowing for targeted pain relief that addresses both symptoms and underlying causes.

Furthermore, when combined with the Y-Age Glutathione and Y-Age Carnosine patches, the Aeon patch takes on a dual role in promoting longevity and reducing signs of aging. This combination can lead to improved cellular health, enhancing not only how one feels but also how one looks. With the ongoing quest for age defiance and wellness, the Aeon patch stands out as a cornerstone of an anti-aging strategy, illuminating the path toward vibrant health.

X39 Stem Cell Patch

Perhaps one of the most revolutionary developments in the LifeWave lineup is the X39 stem cell patch. Touted for its ability to reset genes, this patch facilitates increased energy levels, heightened mental clarity, and improved sports performance. Additionally, it plays a crucial role in recovery, making it an essential tool for athletes and anyone looking to enhance their physical capabilities.

The X39 patch stands at the intersection of science and wellness, tapping into the body's innate healing mechanisms. Its multifaceted benefits extend beyond mere physical enhancement, supporting cognitive function and general vitality. As more individuals turn to stem cell therapy as a means of rejuvenation, the X39 patch offers a non-invasive alternative that integrates seamlessly into daily life.

The LifeWave patches represent a remarkable advancement in phototherapy, each with unique properties that cater to specific health and wellness needs. From boosting fitness and strength with the X49 to enhancing skin health with Alavida, providing anti-inflammatory benefits through Aeon, and activating the body's stem cells with X39, these innovations are paving the way for a new era of holistic health. As you explore these patches, consider how they can be woven into your own wellness journey, unlocking the potential for enhanced healing and vitality.

Future Innovations in LifeWave Technology

As we look toward the future, LifeWave is committed to continuous improvement and innovation. Here are some potential future developments that have been hinted at:

1. **Enhanced Formulations**: One area we can look forward to is the development of enhanced patch formulations. LifeWave has already made strides in creating patches that target various issues, from pain relief to promoting better sleep. In the future, we might see patches that combine multiple benefits into one. Imagine a patch that not only helps with pain but also boosts your energy and enhances your mood all at once!

PATCH TYPE	BENEFITS EXPECTED
Energy Patch	Increased stamina and mental clarity
Sleep Patch	Deep sleep and lucid dreaming
Pain Relief Patch	Targeted relief for chronic pain conditions
Immune Boost Patch	Enhanced immune response and recovery

2. **Smart Technology Integration**: With technology evolving quickly, the integration of smart technology into LifeWave patches is an exciting possibility. Think about patches that could connect to your smartphone via an app. This app could track your usage, monitor your symptoms, and even adjust the patch's effectiveness based on real-time feedback. This would not only give you better control over your wellness journey but also provide valuable data to help LifeWave continue improving their products.

   a) *Usage Tracking:* Monitor how often you wear the patches and for how long.
   b) *Symptom Logging*: Easily keep track of any changes you notice, helping you and your healthcare provider make informed decisions.
   c) *Adjustment Capabilities:* The app could suggest different patches based on your current needs and goals.

3. **Personalized Solutions**: Personalization is a huge trend in health and wellness, and LifeWave could harness this by offering personalized patch recommendations based on your unique needs. Imagine answering a few questions about your lifestyle, health conditions, and wellness goals, and then receiving a customized patch regimen just for you. This tailored approach could lead to more effective results and a better overall experience.

FACTOR	CUSTOMIZATION IDEAS
Health Conditions	Specific patches targeting individual issues
Lifestyle Preferences	Patches suited for athletes vs. sedentary individuals
Age and Gender Considerations	Tailored solutions for different demographic groups

4. **Sustainable Materials**: As the world becomes more eco-conscious, LifeWave might focus on using sustainable materials for their patches. This could include biodegradable materials that maintain the patches' effectiveness while being kinder to the environment. Consumers are increasingly looking for products that reflect their values, and sustainable practices could help LifeWave stand out even more.

   a) *Biodegradable Backing:* Using materials that break down naturally over time.
   b) *Natural Adhesives:* Ensuring that even the adhesives used in patches are eco-friendly.

c) *Recyclable Packaging:* Making sure that the packaging is as sustainable as the patches themselves.

5. **Expanded Research and Collaboration**: Future innovations will likely be driven by ongoing research and collaboration with healthcare professionals. LifeWave may partner with universities, healthcare providers, and wellness experts to conduct studies and gather data on the effectiveness of their patches. This kind of collaboration can lead to new insights and breakthroughs that can enhance the technology behind LifeWave patches.

a) *Long-term Effects:* Studying the cumulative benefits of using patches over an extended period.

b) *Combination Therapies:* Exploring how LifeWave patches work in conjunction with other treatments.

c) *User Experiences:* Gathering feedback from users to continuously improve the product line.

As the technology evolves, so will the education surrounding it. Expect LifeWave to focus on providing more resources, webinars, and community support for users. This could include guides on how to maximize the benefits of the patches and information on the latest research findings.

Combining Patches with Other Therapies

LifeWave patches are designed to promote your body's natural healing processes. They work well on their own, but when combined with other therapies, they can enhance their effects. Whether it's physical therapy, acupuncture, or even good old-fashioned hydration, pairing these methods can help you feel better faster. Here are some great therapies you can consider using alongside LifeWave patches:

Physical Therapy (PT)

Physical therapy is all about helping people recover from injuries, reduce pain, and improve their mobility through exercises and manual techniques. It's commonly used for conditions like back pain, sports injuries, or post-surgery recovery. So, how do LifeWave patches fit into the picture?

LifeWave patches are known for their potential to manage pain and reduce inflammation without any drugs. When you combine PT with the anti-inflammatory benefits of LifeWave patches, the result can be quite impressive. By allowing individuals to experience less pain during PT sessions, the patches can make it easier for them to perform necessary exercises and stretches.

Imagine you're dealing with shoulder pain. If traditional PT is helping but progress is slow due to discomfort during movement, adding LifeWave patches might be beneficial. They could help manage the pain better so you can complete your stretches with less hesitation. This makes PT sessions more productive and can speed up recovery.

Massage Therapy

Who doesn't love a good massage? Massage therapy has long been appreciated for its ability to reduce stress, relieve muscle tension, and promote relaxation. Whether you're dealing with chronic pain or just looking for a way to unwind after a long week, massage can be incredibly beneficial.

Now consider adding LifeWave patches to your massage routine. The calming effects of massage combined with the energy-balancing properties of these patches offer a new level of healing potential. Imagine you're receiving a deep-tissue massage focused on relieving lower back pain. By placing an IceWave patch along the spine or area of discomfort before the session, it may enhance the massage's effects by targeting inflammation directly while promoting healing.

Acupuncture

Acupuncture is a traditional Chinese medicine technique that involves inserting thin needles into specific points on the body. It's known for its effectiveness in alleviating pain and promoting overall wellness. Now, imagine boosting these benefits with LifeWave patches. LifeWave patches work by stimulating the body's own natural healing processes using light (or phototherapy), without any drugs or chemicals.

Combining acupuncture with LifeWave patches can be a powerful way to enhance energy flow throughout the body and provide an extra boost in healing targeted areas. While acupuncture directly works on balancing the body's energy meridians, placing a LifeWave patch near an acupuncture point can continue stimulating that area long after your session ends. This combo approach not only extends the benefits of acupuncture but also aids in pain relief and stress reduction.

Chiropractic Care

Chiropractic care focuses on diagnosing and treating mechanical disorders of the musculoskeletal system, specifically the spine. Chiropractors use hands-on spinal manipulation as well as other alternative treatments to enable the body to heal itself without surgery or medication. Chiropractic adjustments correct alignment issues, alleviate pain, reduce inflammation, and improve the functionality of patients.

Integrating LifeWave patches into chiropractic care is another dynamic duo worth exploring. After a chiropractic adjustment, applying a LifeWave patch to areas where tension or discomfort remains can further reduce pain and inflammation. For example, placing an IceWave patch on sore muscles after a chiropractic session helps in managing pain naturally by aiding muscle relaxation.

Hydration Therapy

Water does not only quench thirst; it is crucial for various bodily functions, including nutrient transport and temperature regulation. When you use LifeWave patches and are well-hydrated, you might notice the patches work more effectively. This happens because proper hydration enhances blood circulation, which in turn can improve the distribution of energy and nutrients throughout your body. By staying hydrated, you might also experience better detoxification processes, allowing your body to flush out toxins more easily.

Now, let's touch base on how to combine this with your LifeWave patches routine. Drink a glass of water before applying the patches. Consider using alkaline or mineral-rich water for added electrolyte balance. Keep a hydration schedule daily—aim for consistency so you can notice the changes in how energetic or rejuvenated you feel when combining these methods regularly.

Essential Oils

Essential oils are concentrated extracts from plants known for their aromatic qualities and potentially beneficial effects on health when used properly. People have been using them for thousands of years for purposes like relaxation, stress relief, and balancing emotions.

Combining essential oils with LifeWave patches can complement each other quite well. For example, if you're using LifeWave patches for stress relief or sleep enhancement, applying lavender or chamomile oil might boost these effects due to their calming properties.

1. **Energy Enhancement (LifeWave Energy Enhancer Patch):** Pair with citrus oils such as orange or lemon for invigorating aromatherapy benefits.

2. **Stress Relief (LifeWave Aeon Patch):** Use with calming oils like lavender or frankincense.

3. **Sleep Support (LifeWave Silent Nights Patch):** Combine with restful scents such as chamomile or ylang-ylang.

When using essential oils with LifeWave patches, consider diffusion methods instead of directly applying them on or near the patch site on your skin to prevent any interference with the patch's adhesive properties or functionality. An oil diffuser necklace or wristband could be handy alternatives as they provide continuous scent throughout your day.

Combining LifeWave Patches with other therapies can be a powerful approach to enhancing wellness. In this chapter, we'll explore how you can integrate LifeWave Patches with meditation, mindfulness, and herbal remedies to maximize their benefits.

Meditation And Mindfulness

Many people find these practices help reduce stress and anxiety, improve emotional health, and enhance their overall sense of well-being. When combined with LifeWave Patches, which are known to support the body's natural healing process through phototherapy, the effects can be amplified. By incorporating patches like Silent Night for better sleep or Aeon for stress reduction during your meditation sessions, you may experience a deeper state of relaxation and a more profound meditative experience.

For example, before starting your meditation or mindfulness practice, apply an Aeon patch and place it on your recommended acupuncture point. As you settle into your practice, focus on the sensations in your body or listen to calming music, allowing the patch to support the reduction of stress and tension naturally. This combination can create a harmonious environment that promotes inner peace and tranquility.

Herbal Remedies

Herbal medicine has been used for centuries to support various aspects of health. Herbs such as chamomile for calming effects, ginger for digestion aid, or ginseng for energy enhancement are quite popular. These natural remedies work by supporting specific body functions or systems which can perfectly complement the benefits provided by LifeWave Patches.

For example, if you're using Energy Enhancer patches during physical activities or workouts, pairing them with herbal teas like ginseng can support sustained energy levels throughout your session. Similarly, using a combination of Y-Age Glutathione patches with herbs known for their antioxidant properties like green tea can intensify detoxification processes in the body.

Tips for Combining Therapies

1. Everyone's response to therapies can differ. Always pay attention to how your body feels and adjust your approach as necessary.
2. If you're unsure about how to combine therapies, it's always a good idea to talk to a healthcare professional. They can provide personalized advice tailored to your needs.
3. If you're new to combining therapies, start with one or two at a time. This way, you can monitor what works best for you without overwhelming yourself.

Expanding Awareness and Accessibility

Many people still don't know about LifeWave patches and the potential benefits they offer. By spreading the word, we can create a community where more individuals can tap into these tools for better health and well-being.

The more you know, the better you can make informed decisions about your health. That's why sharing reliable information about LifeWave patches is important. We can start by hosting workshops, webinars, and local meetups. These events can be casual and fun, allowing people to ask questions, share experiences, and learn more about how to use the patches effectively. Here are some ideas to educate others:

1. **Workshops:** Organize regular sessions where people can come together to learn about the patches. You can demonstrate how to use them, discuss different applications, and share testimonials from users.

2. **Social Media Campaigns:** Use platforms like Instagram, Facebook, and TikTok to share quick tips, success stories, and informative videos about the patches. Engaging content can reach a wider audience and encourage more people to explore their options.

3. **Blogging and Articles:** Write articles on your experiences and findings related to LifeWave patches. You can also invite guest writers to share their stories. This creates a resource hub that people can turn to for information.

Now that we've touched on awareness, let's talk about accessibility. It's great to inform people, but they also need to know where and how to get the patches. Here are some practical ways to increase accessibility:

1. **Local Distributors:** Partner with local health stores or wellness centers to stock LifeWave patches. This makes it easier for people to find and purchase them.

2. **Online Platforms:** Ensure that the online purchasing process is straightforward. Having a user-friendly website makes a big difference. Provide clear information about each patch, its benefits, and how to use it.

3. **Membership Programs:** Consider creating a membership or loyalty program. This could offer discounts or benefits for regular customers, encouraging them to keep using the patches.

4. **Sampling Programs:** Offering samples or trial packs can be a great way to let people experience the patches without a hefty commitment. Once they see the benefits firsthand, they may be more inclined to buy.

Creating a community around LifeWave patches is essential for expanding awareness and accessibility. When people come together around a shared interest, they can support each other, share tips, and celebrate successes. Here are some ways to foster community:

1. **Online Forums:** Create a space where users can share their experiences and ask questions. An online forum or Facebook group can be a supportive environment where everyone feels welcome.

2. **Local Meetups:** Organize casual meetups for patch users. People can come together, share their stories, and even try out different patches together.

3. **Networking with Health Professionals:** Collaborate with healthcare providers who are open to alternative methods. They can help introduce LifeWave patches to their patients, providing an avenue for more individuals to learn about and access these tools.

As we work to expand awareness and accessibility, it's important to measure our impact. Gathering feedback from users can help us understand what's working and what needs improvement. Here's how to track your community outreach efforts:

ACTIVITY	DATE	PARTICIPANTS	FEEDBACK RECEIVED	FOLLOW-UP ACTIONS
Workshop	MM/DD	XX	Positive/Negative	Adjust topics for next session
Social Media Campaign	MM/DD	XX	Engagement Levels	Continue with similar content
Local Distributor Meeting	MM/DD	XX	Interest Level	Explore more partnerships

By keeping track of your initiatives and the feedback you receive, you can fine-tune your approach and maximize the impact of your efforts. Expanding awareness and accessibility around LifeWave patches is a journey we can all be a part of.

CONCLUSION

LifeWave patches offer a natural, drug-free approach to enhancing your health and well-being. By harnessing light to improve energy, reduce pain, enhance sleep, and create a holistic transformation, these small patches pack a powerful punch with their simplicity and effectiveness.

The benefits of LifeWave patches are wide-ranging. From alleviating chronic pain to boosting your overall energy levels, helping you get better rest at night, and even sharpening your mental focus during those pivotal moments of your day – these patches provide an array of positive impacts that contribute significantly to a healthier lifestyle.

With this book, you've discovered how phototherapy can be an integral part of modern wellness practices aimed at maximizing life quality without relying solely on conventional methods. The evidence presented through clinical insights and personal testimonials underscores that LifeWave patches are more than just an alternative; they're an essential addition to your daily health regimen.

Don't let this newfound knowledge gather dust. It's time to take action. Start incorporating LifeWave patches into your routine and embark on your healing journey today. Remember that consistency is key; tracking your progress will provide the motivation you need as you see transformations in your vitality and well-being over time. You now have the tools, so take that first step towards embracing natural health practices.

As we stand at the cusp of advancing technology in natural health solutions, LifeWave patches represent both innovation and accessibility in self-care. The future possibilities for these patches are exciting as research continues to explore new developments in this field. Stayed informed about these updates so you can continue optimizing your approach and outcomes.

Now, it's clear that natural health practices hold significant potential for transformation. When it comes to enhancing our body's innate ability to heal itself, every step taken towards harnessing such techniques contributes not only toward individual wellness but also toward cultivating a broader understanding of holistic health as a society. Thank you for exploring *"The LifeWave Patch Bible"* with us – let's celebrate what photons and good intentions can accomplish together! Now go forth with confidence on this empowering journey towards better living through informed choice-making fueled by nature's intelligence!

APPENDICES

Frequently Asked Questions

1. What are LifeWave patches?

LifeWave patches are small, adhesive patches that you place on your skin. They use a technology called phototherapy to stimulate your body's natural healing processes. The patches contain a mix of organic materials that reflect your body's heat, which can help promote wellness and alleviate discomfort.

2. How do I use the patches?

Using LifeWave patches is super simple! Just clean the area of skin where you want to apply the patch, peel off the backing, and stick it on. It's best to place the patches on areas that are close to where you're feeling discomfort or tension. You can wear them for up to 12 hours at a time, and you can switch them out daily.

3. Are there different types of patches?

Yes, there are several types of LifeWave patches, each designed for specific purposes. Some are aimed at pain relief, while others focus on energy enhancement or promoting better sleep. Make sure to choose the ones that align with your goals, and always read the instructions for optimal placement and use.

4. Can anyone use LifeWave patches?

Generally, yes! LifeWave patches are safe for most people. However, if you are pregnant, nursing, or have a medical condition, it's a good idea to consult with a healthcare professional before using them. Always listen to your body and stop using a patch if you experience any discomfort.

5. How quickly can I expect results?

Results can vary from person to person. Some users notice improvements right away, while others may take a bit longer to feel the effects. It's important to be patient and consistent with your use of the patches. Many people find that regular use helps them experience more significant and lasting benefits over time.

6. Are there any side effects?

LifeWave patches are generally well-tolerated. Most users don't experience side effects, but some might notice mild skin irritation at the application site. If you notice any persistent irritation, it's best to stop using that particular patch and consult a healthcare professional.

7. Can I use the patches while taking medication?

Yes, you can use LifeWave patches alongside most medications. They work on a different principle than pharmaceuticals and should not negatively interact with them. However, it's always wise to speak with a healthcare provider if you have concerns about using patches with your specific medications.

8. How long should I wear the patches?

You can wear LifeWave patches for up to 12 hours at a time. After that, it's a good idea to take a break for at least 12 hours before using a new patch. This allows your skin to breathe and helps ensure optimal effectiveness when you apply a new patch.

9. Can I use multiple patches at once?

Absolutely! Many users find that layering different patches can enhance their effects. Just be mindful of where you place them to avoid skin irritation. Make sure to consult the instructions for each patch type as they may have specific guidelines for use.

10. Where can I buy LifeWave patches?

You can purchase LifeWave patches directly from the official LifeWave website or through authorized distributors. Be cautious of buying from unauthorized sources to ensure you receive genuine products.

11. What if the patches don't work for me?

While many users experience positive results, it's important to remember that everyone's body is different. If you don't see results after consistent use, don't hesitate to reach out to a LifeWave representative or consult a healthcare professional. They can help you explore other options that may be a better fit for your needs.

12. Can children use LifeWave patches?

Yes, LifeWave patches can be used on children, but it's important to consult with a healthcare professional first. They may recommend specific patches or usage guidelines based on the child's age and health condition.

13. Are there specific patches for different ailments?

Absolutely! LifeWave offers various types of patches designed for specific needs, such as pain relief, sleep support, or energy enhancement. Each patch has its own unique benefits, so it's a good idea to explore the options and see which ones resonate with your situation.

14. Do I need to follow a special diet or lifestyle while using the patches?

While there's no strict diet required when using LifeWave patches, maintaining a healthy lifestyle will enhance your overall experience. Eating balanced meals, staying hydrated, and getting regular exercise can help support your body's healing processes.

15. How do I know which patch is right for me?

Choosing the right patch depends on your specific needs and goals. If you're unsure, it can be helpful to read the descriptions and benefits of each patch. You can also consult with a LifeWave distributor or wellness professional who can provide personalized guidance.

16. How do I store my LifeWave patches?

To ensure the longevity of your patches, store them in a cool, dry place, away from direct sunlight and extreme temperatures. Keeping them in their original packaging until you're ready to use them can also help maintain their effectiveness.

Resources for Further Learning

1. **LifeWave Official Website**: The best place to start is the "LifeWave" official website (https://www.lifewave.com). Here, you'll find a wealth of information about the different patches, how they work, and testimonials from people who have experienced amazing results. They also provide updates on new products and research, so bookmark it for easy access!

2. **LifeWave Community Forums**: Join the LifeWave community forums to connect with other users. These forums are a friendly space where you can share experiences, ask questions, and learn from others who are on the same healing journey. Check out "LifeWave Community" to engage with like-minded individuals.

3. **YouTube Channels**: YouTube has a treasure trove of videos about LifeWave patches and phototherapy. Some channels are dedicated to wellness and alternative healing, featuring interviews with experts and testimonials from users. Search for keywords like "LifeWave patches" or "phototherapy" to find content that resonates with you. Just make sure to follow channels that provide credible information!

4. **Books on Holistic Healing**: If you want to expand your understanding of holistic healing, consider reading other books in this genre. Some recommendations include:

   a) *"The Healing Power of Essential Oils" by Eric Zielinski* - This book explores how essential oils can complement your healing journey.
   b) *"The Energy Medicine Kit" by Donna Eden* - It offers insights into energy medicine techniques that can work alongside phototherapy.

These books provide a broader perspective on different healing modalities and can enhance your knowledge.

5. **Podcasts**: Podcasts are a great way to learn while on the go! Look for shows that focus on health, wellness, and alternative therapies. Some popular options include:

   a) *"The Doctor's Farmacy" by Mark Hyman* - He discusses holistic health topics with various experts.

b) *"The Energy Medicine Podcast"* - This show dives into energy healing practices that relate to LifeWave.

Listening to these episodes can give you new insights and inspire you on your wellness journey.

6. **Online Courses and Webinars**: Keep an eye out for online courses or webinars offered by LifeWave or other wellness experts. Many of these opportunities allow you to learn from the comfort of your home and often include Q&A sessions. Check platforms like Udemy or Coursera for relevant courses that can deepen your understanding of healing techniques.

7. **Local Health and Wellness Workshops**: Don't forget to explore local workshops or events in your area. Look for community centers or wellness clinics that host talks or hands-on sessions about phototherapy and holistic health. These in-person gatherings can be great for networking and learning.

8. **Social Media Groups**: Last but not least, consider joining social media groups focused on LifeWave and holistic healing. Facebook and Instagram have communities where users share their experiences, tips, and questions. Just make sure to engage respectfully and verify information before trying anything new.

Recommended Protocols by Condition

Pain Management

Recommended Patches: Ice Wave, Y-Age Aeon

Protocol:

1. Place the Ice Wave patches on the painful area—white patch on the painful spot and the tan patch about 3 inches away.
2. Apply the Y-Age Aeon patch on your wrist (left side for left-handed individuals and right side for right-handed individuals).

Duration: Keep patches on for 12 hours and take them off for 12 hours.

Stress and Anxiety

Recommended Patches: Y-Age Aeon, Silent Nights

Protocol: Apply the Y-Age Aeon patch on the back of your neck and the Silent Nights patch on your wrist.

Duration: Use daily, especially during high-stress situations. Leave on for 12 hours.

Sleep Issues

Recommended Patches: Silent Nights, Y-Age Aeon

Protocol:

1. Place one Silent Nights patch on the bottom of your foot, and another on your wrist.
2. Apply the Y-Age Aeon patch on your abdomen.

Duration: Keep them on for the night to support restful sleep.

Weight Management

Recommended Patches: SP6 Complete, Y-Age Aeon

Protocol:

1. Put the SP6 Complete patch on your left leg, just above the ankle.
2. Place the Y-Age Aeon patch on your wrist.

Duration: Keep the patches on for 12 hours and take them off for 12 hours.

Immune Support

Recommended Patches: Y-Age Aeon, Eon

Protocol: Apply the Y-Age Aeon patch on your left wrist and the Eon patch on your right wrist.

Duration: Use daily for support, keeping them on for 12 hours each day.

Energy Boost

Recommended Patches: Energy Enhancer

Protocol: Place one Energy Enhancer patch on each foot, just below the ball of the foot.

Duration: Wear during the day for an energy boost and remove at night.

Headache Relief

Recommended Patches: Ice Wave, Y-Age Aeon

Protocol:

1. Place the white Ice Wave patch on the site of pain and the tan patch on the opposite side of the body.
2. Apply the Y-Age Aeon patch on your wrist or back of the neck.

Duration: Keep them on for at least 12 hours for maximum effect.

Skin Health

Recommended Patches: Y-Age Aeon, SP6 Complete

Protocol: Use the Y-Age Aeon patch on your abdomen and the SP6 Complete patch on your leg, above the ankle.

Duration: Wear for 12 hours and then take them off for 12 hours.

REFERENCES

[1] Writer, D. S., & Writer, D. S. (2024, July 28). LifeWave: Bringing Wellness to Light - Direct Selling news. Direct Selling News - The News You Need. The Name You Trust. https://www.directsellingnews.com/2024/07/27/lifewave-bringing-wellness-to-light/

[2] Grzybowski, A., Sak, J., & Pawlikowski, J. (2016). A brief report on the history of phototherapy. Clinics in Dermatology, 34(5), 532–537. https://doi.org/10.1016/j.clindermatol.2016.05.002

[3] Gøtzsche PC. Niels Finsen's treatment for lupus vulgaris. J R Soc Med. 2011 Jan;104(1):41-2. doi: 10.1258/jrsm.2010.10k066. PMID: 21205777; PMCID: PMC3014565.

[4] Woodgate P, Jardine LA. Neonatal jaundice: phototherapy. BMJ Clin Evid. 2015 May 22;2015:0319. PMID: 25998618; PMCID: PMC4440981.

[5] Bhms, A. D. (2020, November 3). What light is used in phototherapy for jaundice? MedicineNet. https://www.medicinenet.com/what_light_is_used_in_phototherapy_for_jaundice/article.htm

[6] Campbell PD, Miller AM, Woesner ME. Bright Light Therapy: Seasonal Affective Disorder and Beyond. Einstein J Biol Med. 2017;32:E13-E25. PMID: 31528147; PMCID: PMC6746555.

[7] DermNet. (2023, May 22). UVB phototherapy. DermNet®. https://dermnetnz.org/topics/uvb-phototherapy

[8] Myers E, Kheradmand S, Miller R. An Update on Narrowband Ultraviolet B Therapy for the Treatment of Skin Diseases. Cureus. 2021 Nov 1;13(11):e19182. doi: 10.7759/cureus.19182. PMID: 34873522; PMCID: PMC8634827.

[9] News-Medical. (2019, February 27). PUVA Phototherapy (Psoralen plus UVA). https://www.news-medical.net/health/PUVA-Phototherapy-(Psoralen-plus-UVA).aspx

[10] Bhanjan, A. (2024, April 25). Lighting the Way to Wellness : The science behind LifeWave Technology, X 39, and its impact on neurological HE. Durban Neuro Laser. https://www.durbanneurolaserclinic.co.za/post/lighting-the-way-to-wellness-the-science-behind-lifewave-technology-x-39-and-its-impact-on-neuro

[11] The Science - LifeWave. (n.d.). https://www.lifewave.com/lifewaveinc/home/the-science

[12] Shop all - LifeWave. (n.d.). https://www.lifewave.com/lifewaveinc/store/products

[13] Boost Your Day with LifeWave Energy Enhancer Patches. (n.d.). https://www.lifeandwellness.coach/blog/lifewave-energy-enhancer

[14] Dutch Uncle. (2022, June 21). Healthy Sleep & Silent Nights w David Schmidt LifeWave 27 Jan, 2021 [Video]. YouTube. https://www.youtube.com/watch?v=IgEqHb9bxEQ

[15] Kimberly. (2024, August 14). What are lifewave patches? | Article | JUST SKIN CLINIC. JUST SKIN CLINIC. https://justskinclinic.co.za/what-are-lifewave-patches/

[16] Graham, M. (2024, October 15). Avoid these common mistakes when using Lifewave patches — Megan Graham Beauty and Lifestyle | Lifewave Brand Partner. Megan Graham Beauty and Lifestyle | Lifewave Brand Partner. https://www.megangrahambeauty.com/blog/avoid-these-common-mistakes-when-using-lifewave-patches

[17] Piven, E., Dharia, R., Jones, K., Davis, C., & Nazeran, H. (2013). Effect of IceWave®organic nanoscale patches on reduction of musculoskeletal pain. TANG [HUMANITAS MEDICINE], 3(1), 5.1-5.5. https://doi.org/10.5667/tang.2012.0037

[18] Silent Nights Patches - LifeWave. (n.d.). https://lifewave.com/lifewaveinc/store/product/32001.029.001

[19] Homer, N. (2015). A double-blind placebo-controlled heart rate variability investigation to evaluate the quantitative effects of the organic nanoscale aeon patch on the autonomic nervous system. CELLMED, 5(1), 5-5, https://doi.org/10.5667/tang.2014.0024

[20] ECHAD HARMONY. (2024, November 12). Mike Tyson trains with lifewave technology [Video]. YouTube. https://www.youtube.com/watch?v=ZfWMK4nW89c